Ethics Manual

Approved by the
American College of Physicians

Third Edition

ACP Ethics Committee
Edwin P. Maynard, MD, Chair; Karen Coblens, MD; Errol D. Crook, MD; Lee Dunn, Jr., JD, LLM; Arthur W. Feinberg, MD; Lloyd W. Kitchens, Jr., MD; Bernard Lo, MD; William A. Reynolds, MD; Gerald E. Thomson, MD; and Susan W. Tolle, MD

Published by the American College of Physicians
Philadelphia, Pennsylvania

Third Edition

Printed in the United States of America

Reprinted from *Annals of Internal Medicine*. 1992;117:947-960; and from *ACP Observer*, October 1990; February 1991; September 1991; November 1991; and July 1992.

Library of Congress Cataloging-in-Publication Data

American College of Physicians. Ad Hoc Committee on Medical Ethics.
American College of Physicians ethics manual / American College of Physicians Ethics Committee.—3rd ed.
68 pp. cm.
"Reprinted from Annals of internal medicine, 1992: 117-947-960: and from ACP observer, October 1990: February 1991: September 1991: November 1991: and July 1992" — T.p. verso.
Includes bibliographical references.
ISBN 0-943126-26-6 : $12.00 (10.00 ACP member)
1. Medical ethics. I. Title. II. Title: Ethics manual.
[DNLM: 1. Ethics, Medical—Collected works. W 50 A506a 1991a]
R724.A59 1993
174'.2—dc20
DNLM/DLC
for Library of Congress 92-48551
CIP

Table of Contents

Medicine, law, and social values are not static and must be re-examined periodically. This edition of the ACP Ethics Manual *covers emerging issues in medical ethics and revisits some old issues. The overview of the evolution of medical ethics, which appeared in previous editions of the* Manual, *has been eliminated to allow more space for the consideration of today's ethical dilemmas. Other changes include a revised chapter on end-of-life care, discussion of physician-assisted suicide, revised sections on conflicts of interest and on medical risk to the physician and patient, given developments in human immunodeficiency virus (HIV) infection and the acquired immunodeficiency syndrome (AIDS), and discussion of sexual contact between physician and patient. A statement on disclosure of errors and a section on care of the physician's family have also been added. The sections on confidential information told by a patient's family or friend to the physician; on physician-pharmaceutical industry relations; on physicians in training; and on the impaired physician have been expanded. Sections on advertising, peer review, and resource allocation have been revised. The literature of biomedical ethics expands at a rate that does not allow a bibliography to remain current, so an exhaustive list of references or suggested readings is not included in this manual. Instead, only cited references are listed.*

The *ACP Ethics Manual* is designed to facilitate the process of making ethical decisions in clinical practice and medical research. Because ethics must be understood within a historical and cultural context, the second edition of the *Manual* included a brief overview of the cultural, philosophical, and religious underpinnings of modern medical ethics. In this third edition, we refer the reader to that overview (1) and to other sources (2-5) that more fully explore the rich heritage of medical ethics.

Members of the Ethics Committee for the 1991-92 term who developed this third edition of the manual were Edwin P. Maynard, MD, *Chair*; Karen Coblens, MD; Errol D. Crook, MD; Lee Dunn, Jr., JD, LLM; Arthur W. Feinberg, MD; Lloyd W. Kitchens, Jr., MD; Bernard Lo, MD; William A. Reynolds, MD; Gerald E. Thomson, MD; and Susan W. Tolle, MD. Staff editors were Lois Snyder, JD, and Janet Weiner, MPH. Additional staff contributions were made by H. Denman Scott, MD (Senior Vice President, Health and Public Policy), Linda Johnson White (Director, Department of Scientific Policy), and Linda J. Sowers. Approved by the Board of Regents on 10 July 1992.

The *Manual* raises ethical issues and presents general guidelines. In applying these guidelines, physicians should consider individual circumstances and use their best judgment. Physicians are morally as well as legally accountable, and the two may not be concordant. Segregation and slavery, for example, were once legal in this country but are never morally defensible. Physicians must keep in mind the distinctions and potential conflicts between legal and ethical obligations when making clinical decisions and must seek counsel when concerned about the potential legal consequences of ethical decisions. We refer to the law in this manual for illustrative purposes only; these references should not be taken as a statement of the law, which can vary from state to state, or of the legal consequences of a physician's actions.

The law does not always establish positive duties (what one should do) to the extent that professional (especially medical) ethics does. Our current understanding of medical ethics is based on the principles from which these positive duties emerge. The relative value of such principles, and conflicts among them, often account for the ethical dilemmas physicians face.

These principles include beneficence—the duty to promote good and prevent harm to patients; nonmaleficence—the duty to do no harm to patients; and respect for a patient's autonomy—the duty to protect and foster an individual's free and uncoerced choices (6). From the principle of respect for autonomy are also derived the rules for truth-telling, disclosure, and informed consent.

In addition, considerations of justice guide the physician's role as citizen and in societal decisions about resource allocations. The principle of distributive justice demands that we seek the morally correct distribution of benefits and burdens in society. Determining that distribution, especially when allocating resources to health care, is the focus of intense debate in our society. More than ever, concerns about justice challenge the traditional role of physician as patient advocate.

A broad consensus is emerging that the U.S. health care system does not serve all of its citizens well and that major reform is needed. Any such reform, constrained by growing concerns that our resources are limited, faces important issues of priority and equity. Health care costs will be a major focus, and our society's values will be tested in decisions about resource allocations.

These issues attract widespread public attention, and their debate is covered regularly in the press. Increasingly, government, through legislation, administrative action, or judicial decision, is involved in medical ethics. It is crucial that a responsible physician perspective be heard as these societal decisions are made.

The decision to update this manual was prompted by the continued emergence of complex ethical issues not addressed in previous editions. From genetic testing before conception to dilemmas at the end of life, physicians, with patients and families, are called on to make difficult ethical decisions. The 1970s saw the development of bioethics as a field, followed by a series of reports by the President's Commission for the Study of Ethical Problems in Medicine and Biomedical and Behavioral Research on important issues such as informed consent (7, 8), access to health care (9), genetic screening and engineering (10, 11), and foregoing life-sustaining treatment (12, 13). These and other modern dilemmas such as AIDS, physician-assisted suicide, and the physician as entrepreneur challenge us to reconsider basic principles regarding confidentiality, decisions to limit treatment, and the nature of the patient-physician relationship.

Today, the convergence of various forces—scientific advances, public education, the civil rights and consumer movements, the effects of law and economics on medicine, and the moral heterogeneity of our society—demands that we as physicians clearly articulate the ethical principles that guide our behavior, whether in clinical care, in research, or as citizens.

The ACP Ethics Committee, composed of practicing internists, medical ethicists, and educators, wrote this manual for our colleagues in medicine, but it will also serve as a reference for others seeking ACP positions on ethical issues. In addition, we hope this manual will stimulate reasoned debate and widen the area of agreement on medical ethics. Such a debate may also stimulate critical evaluation and discussion of law and public policy regarding the difficult ethical issues facing patients and physicians.

The Physician and the Patient

The patient's welfare and best interests must be the physician's main concern. The physician should treat and cure when possible and help patients cope with illness, disability, and death. In all instances, the physician must help maintain the dignity of the person and respect the uniqueness of each person.

The interests of the patient should always be promoted, whether care occurs under the auspices of fee-for-service, health maintenance organization, preferred provider organization, the Armed Forces, the Department of Veterans Affairs, or publicly supported medical facilities or whether the patient is mentally competent, incompetent, permanently unconscious, chronically or acutely ill, or a minor or an elderly person. The physician's obligations to the patient remain unchanged even though the patient-physician relationship may be affected by the health care delivery system or the patient's state.

Whatever the treatment setting, at the beginning of a relationship the physician must understand the patient's complaints and underlying feelings and expectations. After they agree on the problem before them, the physician presents one or more courses of action. If both parties agree, the patient may then authorize the physician to initiate a course of action, and the physician accepts this responsibility. The relationship has mutual obligations: The physician must be professionally competent, act responsibly, and treat the patient with compassion and respect. The patient should understand and consent to the treatment and should participate responsibly in the care. Although the physician deserves fair compensation for services rendered, professionalism and a sense of duty to the patient and to society should take precedence over concern about compensation; the physician's primary commitment is to the patient.

Physicians and patients may have different concepts of the meaning and resolution of medical problems. The care of the patient and satisfaction of both parties are best served if the physician and patient discuss their expectations and concerns openly. The physician must be flexible and open to compromise to address the patient's concerns. The physician cannot be required to violate fundamental personal values, standards of scientific or ethical practice, or the law. There are occasions when the patient's beliefs—religious, cultural, or otherwise—dictate decisions that run counter to medical advice. The physician is obliged to try to understand clearly the beliefs and the viewpoints of the patient. After a serious attempt to resolve differences, if the physician is unable to carry out the patient's wishes, the physician must withdraw and transfer care of the patient.

Initiating and Discontinuing the Treatment Relationship

By history, tradition, and professional oath, physicians have a moral obligation to provide care to the sick. Although this is a collective obligation, each physician is required to do his or her fair share to ensure that all sick people receive adequate treatment. An individual patient-physician relationship is based on mutual agreement regarding medical care for the patient. A physician may not discriminate against a class or category of patients but, in the absence of a preexisting relationship, is not ethically obliged to provide care to an individual person unless no other physician is available, as in some isolated communities; emergency treatment is required, under which circumstances the physician is morally bound to provide care and, if necessary, to arrange for proper follow-up; or a previous contractual obligation exists.

A patient is free to change physicians and is entitled to the information contained in the medical records. Under exceptional circumstances, the physician may discontinue the professional relationship by notifying the patient and, with the approval of the patient, transferring to another physician the information in the record, provided adequate care is available elsewhere and the patient's health is not jeopardized in the process. Continuity of care must be assured to the best of the physician's ability. Physician-initiated termination is a serious event and should be undertaken only after genuine attempts to understand and resolve differences.

Confidentiality

Confidentiality is a fundamental tenet of medical care. Confidentiality respects the privacy of patients, encourages them to seek medical care and discuss their problems candidly, and prevents discrimination based on their medical condition. The physician must not release information without the patient's consent, unless required by the law or if there is a duty to warn another. Confidentiality, like other ethical duties, is not absolute. It may have to be overridden to protect others or the public—for example, to warn sexual partners that a patient has syphilis or is infected with HIV. Before breaching confidentiality, the physician should make every effort to discuss the issues with the patient. If it is necessary to breach confidentiality, it should be done in a way that minimizes harm to the patient.

Confidentiality is increasingly hard to maintain in this era of computerized record keeping and electronic data processing, the faxing of patient information, third-party payment for medical services, and the sharing of patient care among numerous medical professionals and institutions. Physicians should be aware of the increased risk for invasion of patients' privacy. Also, within their own institutions, physicians should advocate policies and procedures to secure the confidentiality of patient records.

In the care of the adolescent patient, family support is important. However, it must be balanced with confidentiality and respect for the adolescent's autonomy in health care decisions and in relationships with health care providers (14). Physicians should be knowledgeable about state laws governing the right of adolescent patients to confidentiality and the adolescent's legal right to consent to treatment.

Occasionally, the physician receives information from a patient's friends or relatives and is asked to withhold the source of that information from the patient (15). The physician is not obliged to keep such "secrets" from the patient. The informant should be urged to address the patient directly and to encourage the patient to discuss the information with the physician. The physician should use sensitivity and judgment in deciding whether to use the information and whether to reveal its source to the patient. The physician should always act in the best interests of the patient.

The discussion of the problems of an identified patient by professional staff in public places (for example, in elevators) violates confidentiality and is unethical. Outside of an educational setting, even discussions of an unidentified patient in front of others not involved in that patient's care are unwise and impair the public's confidence in the medical profession. Likewise, confidentiality must be maintained for patients who are well known to the public. Physicians of public figures should remember that they are not free to discuss or disclose information about a patient's health without the explicit consent of the patient.

The Patient and the Medical Record

Ethically and legally, patients have the right to know what is in their medical records. Legally, the actual chart is the property of the physician or institution, although the information in the chart is the property of the patient. Most states have laws that guarantee the patient personal access to the medical record. The physician may exercise some discretion in deciding how information in the chart should be provided, but the physician must release information to the patient or to a third party at the request of the patient. Physicians should retain the original of the chart and radiographic studies, responding to a patient's request with copies unless the original record is required by law. To protect confidentiality, information should only be released with the written permission of the patient or the patient's legally authorized representative.

Consent

The physician is obligated to ensure that the patient or, where appropriate, the surrogate be adequately informed about the nature of the patient's medical condition, the objectives of proposed treatment, treatment alternatives, possible outcomes, and the risks involved.

The doctrine of informed consent goes beyond the question of whether consent was given for a treatment or intervention. Rather, it focuses on the content of that consent. The physician is required to provide enough information to allow a patient to make an informed judgment about how to proceed. The physician's presentation should be understandable to the patient, should be unbiased, and should include the physician's recommendation. The patient's (or surrogate's) concurrence must be free and uncoerced.

In most medical encounters, when the patient presents to a physician for evaluation and care, consent can be presumed. The underlying condition and treatment options are explained to the patient, and treatment is rendered and not refused. In medical emergencies, consent to treatment necessary to maintain life or restore health can generally be implied, unless it is known that the patient would refuse the intervention.

Expressed consent most often occurs in the hospital setting where written or oral consent is given for a particular procedure. Legal criteria for informed consent vary from state to state, and physicians should know the law in the jurisdiction in which they practice.

All adult patients are considered competent to make decisions about medical care unless a court declares them incompetent. In clinical practice, however, physicians and family members usually make decisions for patients who lack decision making capacity, without a formal competency hearing in the courts. This clinical approach can be ethically justified if the physician has carefully determined that the patient is incapable of understanding the nature of the proposed treatment, the alternatives, the risks and benefits, and the consequences.

When a patient lacks decision making capacity, an appropriate surrogate should make decisions with the physician. Ideally, surrogate decision-makers should know the patient's choices and values and act in the best interests of the patient. If the patient has designated a proxy, as through a durable power of attorney for health care, that choice should be respected. When patients have not selected surrogates, standard clinical practice is for family members to serve as surrogates. Some states designate the order in which family members will serve as surrogates, and physicians should be aware of legal requirements in their state for surrogate appointment and decision making. In some cases, all parties may agree that a close friend is a more appropriate surrogate than a relative.

Physicians should take reasonable care to assure that the surrogate's decisions are consistent with the patient's preferences and best interests. When possible, these decisions should be reached in the medical setting by physicians, appropriate surrogates, and other caregivers. Physicians should emphasize that decisions be based on what the patient would want and not on what surrogates would choose for themselves. If disagreements cannot be resolved, hospital ethics committees may be helpful. Courts should be used as a last resort, when other processes fail or as required by state law.

Physicians should obtain consent from the patient for the disposal and use of tissue, organs, or other body parts removed during diagnostic or operative procedures. With the goal of respecting the wishes and values of the deceased, the opportunity to donate organs should be considered by surrogates and consent obtained, in accordance with state law, to use organs and tissues for transplantation or research.

Disclosure

The patient must be well informed in order to make health care decisions and work intelligently in partnership with the physician. Effective patient-physician communication can dispel uncertainty and fear and enhance healing and patient satisfaction.

Information should be given in terms the patient can understand. The physician should be sensitive to the patient's responses in setting the pace of disclosure, particularly when the illness is very serious. Disclosure should never be a mechanical or perfunctory process. Upsetting news and information should be presented to the patient in a way that minimizes distress. If the patient is unable to comprehend, then the patient's condition should be fully disclosed to an appropriate surrogate.

In general, disclosure to patients is a fundamental ethical requirement. However, society recognizes the "therapeutic privilege," which is an exemption from detailed disclosure when such disclosure has a high likelihood of causing serious and irreversible harm to the patient. On balance, this privilege should be interpreted narrowly; invoking it too broadly can undermine the entire concept of informed consent.

In addition, physicians should disclose to patients information about procedural or judgment errors made in the course of care, if such information significantly affects the care of the patient. Errors do not necessarily constitute improper, negligent, or unethical behavior.

Decisions about Reproduction

The ethical duty to disclose relevant information about reproduction to the patient may conflict with the physician's personal moral standards regarding abortion, sterilization, or contraception. A physician who objects to abortion on moral, religious, or ethical grounds need not become involved, either by offering advice to the patient or by involvement in the surgical procedure. As in any other medical situation, the physician does have a duty to assure that the patient is offered information on the full range of options from a qualified colleague. This duty applies to issues of sterilization and contraception as well.

Social, political, and religious beliefs have extended the issue of abortion beyond medical considerations. Physicians must be familiar with the law relating to abortion in their locales.

If a patient who is a minor requests termination of pregnancy without her parent's knowledge, the physician should attempt to persuade her of the benefits of having her parents involved. If unsuccessful, or if parental involvement would be harmful, the physician may have a conflict between the ethical duty to maintain confidentiality and the physician's legal responsibility to the patient's parents or guardian. In such cases, the physician should seek counsel regarding the specific requirements of state and federal law and should be guided by his or her conscience in light of the law.

Medical Risk to the Physician and Patient

It is unethical for a physician to refuse to care for a patient solely because of medical risk, or perceived risk, to the physician. Traditionally, the ethical imperative for physicians to provide care has overridden risk to the treating physician, even during epidemics. In recent decades, with better control of such risks, physicians have practiced medicine in the absence of risk as a prominent concern. However, the appearance of AIDS necessitates reaffirmation of the ethical imperative (16).

Because HIV can be transmitted from patient to physician, some physicians avoid the care of HIV-infected patients. Physicians and hospitals are obligated to provide competent and humane care to all patients, including those with HIV infection. The denial of appropriate care to a class of patients for any reason is unethical (17).

Transmission of HIV from physician to patient is possible, although the risk is so extraordinarily low that it cannot be measured. Physicians should evaluate their risk for HIV exposure, both in their personal lives and in the workplace. Physicians who may have been exposed have an ethical obligation to be tested for HIV and other blood-borne pathogens and should do so voluntarily. Seropositive physicians should place themselves under the guidance of a local expert review panel, which will determine in a confidential manner whether practice restrictions are appropriate based on the physician's compliance with infection control precautions and physical and mental fitness to work. Infection with HIV does not in itself justify restrictions on the practice of an otherwise competent health care worker.

Physicians have several obligations regarding nosocomial risk for HIV infection. Physicians should help the public understand the low level of this risk and put it in the perspective of other medical risks, while acknowledging public concern. Physicians provide medical care to health care workers. Part of such care is discussing with health care workers their ethical obligation to know their risk for HIV, to voluntarily seek HIV testing if they are at risk, and to take reasonable steps to protect patients. The physician who is caring for a seropositive health care worker needs to evaluate the health care worker's fitness to work. In some cases, seropositive health care workers cannot be persuaded to comply with accepted infection control guidelines, or impaired physicians cannot be persuaded to restrict their practice. In such exceptional cases, the treating physician may need to breach confidentiality and report to appropriate authorities in order to protect patients and maintain public trust in the profession, even though such actions might have legal consequences.

The Physician and Unorthodox Treatments

Requests by patients for treatment outside the recognized methods of medical care pit the physician's judgment on optimal medical therapy against the patient's acknowledged right to choose what care to receive and from whom. Such a request warrants the physician's careful attention. Before advising a patient, the physician should become familiar with the care being considered and should ascertain the reason for the request, for example, whether it stems from dissatisfaction with current care or from claims made about the unorthodox treatment. Next, as with the process of informed consent, the physician should be sure that the patient understands the condition, traditional medical treatment, and expected outcomes. The physician should discuss realistically and dispassionately with the patient what can be expected from different methods of care. The physician should not abandon the patient who elects to try an unorthodox treatment and should regard the patient's decision with grace and compassion. In general, the physician should not participate in such treatment. When the treatment is clearly harmful to patients, the physician should seek the best means by which to protect the patient and, where possible, have the dangerous therapy challenged.

Care of the Physician's Family

Physicians should be discouraged from treating close friends or members of their own families. Although many physicians do treat family members, some report great discomfort when doing so (18). Potential problems include feelings of constraints on time or resources, incomplete disclosure of patient information, or limited physical examination. The physician's emotional proximity can result in a loss of objectivity. If a physician does treat a close friend or family member out of necessity, the patient should be transferred to another physician as soon as is practical. Physicians should encourage all friends and family members to have their own personal physician.

Sexual Contact between Physician and Patient

It is unethical for a physician to become sexually involved with a current patient even if the patient initiates or consents to the contact. Issues of dependency, trust, transference, and inequalities of power lead to increased vulnerability of the patient and require that a physician not cross the boundary.

Even sexual involvement between physicians and former patients raises concern. The impact of the patient-physician relationship may be viewed very differently by physicians and former patients, and either may underestimate the influence of the past professional relationship. Many former patients continue to feel dependency and transference toward their physician long after the professional relationship has ended. The intense trust often established between physician and patient raises similar concerns about ongoing patient vulnerability in a subsequent sexual relationship. A sexual relationship with a former patient is unethical if the physician "uses or exploits the trust, knowledge, emotions or influence derived from the previous professional relationship" (19). Because it may be difficult for the physician to judge this influence, we advise consultation with a colleague or other professional before becoming sexually involved with a former patient.

Financial Arrangements

Financial relationships between patients and physicians vary from fee-for-service, to government contractual arrangements, to prepaid insurance. At the beginning of patient-physician contact, it is important for patients to have a general knowledge of physician fees and the probable overall costs of medical care. Financial arrangements should be clarified and means of payment or inability to pay should be established. Once the patient-physician relationship has been established by mutual agreement, the physician's duty is to see that appropriate care is rendered, unless the relationship is discontinued. Fees for physician services should accurately reflect the services provided.

When physicians elect to offer a colleague "professional courtesy" (care at no charge or at a reduced fee), such care must be of the same quality provided other patients, regardless of the financial arrangements. In such situations, physicians and patients should function without feelings of constraints on time or resources and without short-cut approaches. Colleague-patients who initiate questions in informal settings put the treating physician in a less than ideal position to provide optimal care. Both parties should prevent such inappropriate practice.

As professionals dedicated to serving the sick, physicians should contribute services to the uninsured and underinsured and do their fair share to ensure that all people receive adequate medical care.

Conflicts of Interest

When conflicts arise, the moral principle is clear. The welfare of the patient must at all times be paramount, and the physician must insist that the medically appropriate level of care take primacy over fiscal considerations imposed by the physician's own practice, investments, or financial arrangements. Trust in the profession is undermined when there is even the appearance of impropriety.

Potential influences on clinical judgment cover a wide range, including financial incentives inherent in the practice environment (such as incentives to overutilize in the fee-for-service setting or underutilize in the managed care setting [20]), drug industry gifts, and business arrangements involving referrals. Physicians must be conscious of all potential influences, and their actions should be guided by appropriate utilization and not by other factors.

Physicians should avoid any business arrangement that might lead to personal gain influencing their decisions in the care of the patient. In general, physicians should not refer patients to an outside facility in which they have invested and at which they do not directly provide care or services (21).

An exception to this general rule recognizes that investments in or ownership of health care facilities by physicians who refer to such facilities is appropriate when capital funding and necessary services are provided that would otherwise not be made available. In such a situation, in addition to disclosing these interests to patients, there must be safeguards against both abuse and even the appearance of impropriety (21).

Investments in publicly traded securities (stocks, bonds) do not represent conflicts of interest as long as ownership does not influence decisions or actions in the care of patients. There is also no objection to a physician being engaged in any legitimate business activity unrelated to medical practice that does not compromise patient care.

The acceptance of gifts, hospitality, trips, and subsidies of all types from medical equipment or pharmaceutical companies is strongly discouraged. The increasing sophistication of marketing techniques places the physician in situations where clinical judgment may be affected and where the perception, as well as the reality, of a conflict of interest is heightened (22). Therefore, work-related gifts of minimal value such as pens or notepads might be acceptable, whereas cash gifts or payment for enrolling patients in studies would be unacceptable. In addition to following the Royal College of Physicians guideline, "Would I be willing to have this arrangement generally known?" (23), physicians should ask, "What would the public or my patients think of this arrangement?"

Other potential conflicts can arise in continuing medical education and in publishing. Physicians must evaluate and correct for any bias in interpreting medical information provided by detail persons, advertising, or industry-sponsored educational programs. Physicians with ties to a particular company should disclose their interests when speaking or writing about a company product. Most journal editors require that authors and peer reviewers disclose any potential conflicts of interest. Editors themselves should be free from conflicts of interest regarding particular papers.

Advertising

Advertising by physicians is unethical when it contains statements that are unsubstantiated, false, deceptive, or misleading, including statements that mislead by omitting necessary information.

Fee Splitting

A physician's professional fees should be received for the services rendered directly to a patient. A fee paid one physician by another for the referral of a patient is unethical. It is also unethical for a physician to receive a commission or "kickback" from anyone, including a company that manufactures or sells medical instruments or medications that may be used in the care of patients.

Decisions Near the End of Life

Decisions near the end of life have a clinical and psychological intensity that distinguishes them from more routine clinical encounters. Although this section highlights some of the special features of end-of-life decision making, the central point to remember is that the basic principles of informed consent, shared decision making, and the use of surrogate decision-makers when necessary, described elsewhere in this manual, apply also to end-of-life decisions.

Who Should Make the Decision?

Patients who have decision making capacity and who are adequately informed of their clinical situation and options have the right to refuse any recommended medical treatment, including life-sustaining treatment, except in rare circumstances when the law forces a patient to accept treatment. The patient's right is based on the philosophical concept of autonomy, the common law right of self-determination, and the patient's liberty interest under the Constitution in refusing unwanted medical care. The crux of the issue is that the patient's (rather than the physician's) assessment of the benefits and burdens of treatment should determine what treatment is administered or withheld.

Many patients, particularly those with terminal or irreversible illness, elect to forego life-sustaining treatments.

In some cases, physicians may consider such refusals of treatment unwise. Physicians have an obligation to ensure that the refusal is truly informed, to give a clear recommendation, and to try to persuade the patient, but ultimately they must accept the patient's decision.

When patients lack decision making capacity (*see* "Consent"), decisions regarding life-sustaining treatment may be complicated for several reasons: Standards for assessing decision making capacity may be unclear; the criteria for making decisions for such patients may be controversial; and disagreement may occur about who is the appropriate surrogate decision-maker.

Criteria for Decisions

In order of priority, decisions should be based on advance directives, substituted judgments, and the best interests of the patient.

Patients' informed goals and choices should be respected even if they no longer have decision making capacity. Through *advance directives*, competent patients state what treatments they would accept or decline if they lost decision making capacity. In giving advance directives, patients should also indicate their general goals for care and their choice of surrogate.

Oral statements to family members, friends, and health care professionals are the most common form of advance directive. However, oral statements are problematic if they are vague and ambiguous or if they were casual comments rather than seriously intended directives. Because some states regard oral advance directives as untrustworthy, written advance directives have several advantages. Living wills can have a narrow scope of application, in most states providing guidance only for terminal conditions, the definition of which varies; they may not apply to patients in a persistent vegetative state. Living wills generally are limited to the refusal of interventions that would only prolong the process of dying. Some states explicitly exclude intravenous fluids and tube feedings from the interventions that may be refused, although courts might rule that such an exclusion violates patient rights.

The durable power of attorney for health care can be more comprehensive and flexible than the living will; the patient appoints a surrogate (also called an agent) to make decisions if the patient becomes unable to do so. The surrogate is required to act in accordance with the patient's previously expressed preferences or best interests. Patients can usually indicate specific treatments they would accept or refuse in various situations. Different states have specific procedures for appointing surrogates; some have durable power of attorney for health care or health care proxy laws for the appointment of surrogates, whereas others allow appointment as part of living wills. Physicians need to be familiar with state laws. Copies of written advance directives should be placed in the patient's medical record.

Physicians should raise the issue of advance directives routinely with competent adult patients in outpatient visits and encourage them to provide advance directives and to discuss their preferences with their surrogate and family members. In addition, the Patient Self-Determination Act of 1990 requires hospitals, nursing homes, health maintenance organizations, and hospices that participate in Medicare and Medicaid programs to provide patients, on admission or enrollment, with information about their right to provide advance directives. These health care institutions are required to respect advance directives to the fullest extent permitted under state law. Discussions between physicians and patients let the physician know the patient's preferences and values, enable physicians to check that choices are informed and up-to-date, and reassure patients that the physician is willing to discuss these sensitive issues and will respect their choices. Discussions about patient preferences should be documented in the medical record.

Two standards have been developed for surrogate decision making in cases where the patient has not left an advance directive. In a *substituted judgment*, the surrogate attempts to make the judgment that the patient, if competent, would have made. This approach is feasible and desirable when the surrogate knows the patient's goals, values, and choices.

If the patient's values and preferences are unknown or unclear, decisions should be based on the patient's *best interests*. In making decisions about their care, patients often take into account their current and projected quality of life. For patients who lack decision making capacity, quality of life may also be an integral aspect of their best interests. Assessments of quality of life according to the patient's perspective and values should be respected. Quality-of-life judgments made by a person not familiar with the patient's perspective should be suspect. Because family members and health care workers may project their own values onto the incapacitated patient, there is a significant risk of bias and discrimination. In the current medical environment, which emphasizes cost containment, physicians should not use quality-of-life standards that may lead to various groups of patients being denied appropriate treatments.

Dilemmas Regarding Life-Sustaining Treatments

WITHDRAWING OR WITHHOLDING TREATMENT

The same reasons that justify not starting treatment also justify stopping treatment. Indeed, the reasons for withdrawing a treatment may be more compelling, because it may have proved unsuccessful or because the patient's prognosis and wishes may have been clarified. Treatments should not be withheld solely for fear that if started they cannot be withdrawn, because patients may be denied potentially beneficial therapies. Time-limited trials of therapy may establish the patient's prognosis. Court rulings and most ethicists have found no legal or ethical difference between withdrawing and withholding treatment. Nonetheless, some health care workers or family members may have a visceral reluctance to withdraw treatments. Physicians need to be sensitive to such emotional reactions. Usually, explicit discussion of such feelings resolves disagreements. If no agreement is reached, physicians must keep in mind that the patient has a right to refuse treatment and arrange for a transfer of care if necessary.

DO-NOT-RESUSCITATE ORDERS

Cardiopulmonary resuscitation may be effective in reversing unexpected sudden death. However, it is not appropriate for every patient who has cardiopulmonary arrest, particularly a patient with terminal irreversible illness whose death is expected. Resuscitation is an emergency treatment that must be applied immediately to be successful. Because there is no time during a cardiopulmonary arrest for deliberation and decision making, decisions about resuscitation should be made before a clinical crisis occurs.

Physicians should invite all seriously ill patients or their surrogates to discuss resuscitation. Such discussions often lead to a comprehensive plan for care. The physician must consider both the medical indications and the patient's preferences. Like other life-sustaining interventions, resuscitation may be withheld if informed patients or appropriate surrogates so choose.

In some cases, after discussions with the physician, a patient or surrogate continues to insist on resuscitation, even though the physician believes that it would be futile. Futility, as it pertains to resuscitation, has been defined to apply to either its initial failure to restore circulation and breathing or to the subsequent failure to discharge the patient alive from the hospital. It is appropriate for physicians to write a do-not-resuscitate (DNR) order when resuscitation would not restore circulation and breathing—for example, in progressive multisystem organ failure. It is more controversial whether it is appropriate for physicians to write a unilateral DNR order in situations where discharge alive after resuscitation would be unprecedented. The physician should make every effort to ensure that misunderstanding, poor communication, or unaddressed psychosocial concerns are not the reasons for an apparently irrational insistence on resuscitation. If physicians write a unilateral DNR order, they must inform the patient or surrogate. If DNR orders are not written, it is unethical for physicians and nurses to perform half-hearted resuscitation efforts (so-called "slow codes").

The DNR order should be written in the medical record. In some institutions, the term "no CPR" is used to emphasize that a decision to withhold resuscitation does not imply that other interventions should be withheld or withdrawn. However, when DNR orders are discussed, the physician should also discuss with the patient or surrogate, housestaff, and nursing staff the overall goals and specific plans for care. It is essential that patients or surrogates understand that a DNR order does not mean that the patient will be abandoned.

TERMINALLY ILL PATIENTS

In this manual, we consider terminally ill patients as those whose condition is irreversible whether treated or not and who most likely will die within 3 to 6 months. The general guidelines for shared decision making regarding life-sustaining treatment also apply in terminal illness. Although the underlying disease cannot be reversed, the physician must work closely with the patient to make the patient as comfortable as possible by reducing physical pain and psychological suffering. Palliative care (as emphasized by the hospice concept) includes pain relief, psychological and social support, and possibly surgery, radiation, and antibiotic therapy if they will make the patient more comfortable. The physician should also help provide support to the patient's family, friends, and other care providers.

DETERMINATION OF DEATH

Death of the entire brain, including the brain stem, is now an accepted standard in all the states for determining death when the use of cardiopulmonary life support precludes the use of traditional criteria.

When clinically appropriate, physicians should offer the next of kin or surrogate the opportunity to donate the patient's organs for transplantation. After a patient has been declared dead by brain death criteria, life support should be discontinued. There may be circumstances, such as the need to preserve organs for transplantation, to counsel and comfort the bereaved, or to sustain a viable fetus, in which physicians may elect to support bodily functions temporarily after death of the whole brain has been established.

IRREVERSIBLE LOSS OF CONSCIOUSNESS

Discontinuing life support for persons who are permanently unconscious or in a persistent vegetative state remains controversial when the patient's preferences are not known. Such patients are not terminally ill or brain dead, but they lack awareness of their surroundings and the ability to respond purposefully to them. The current legal and ethical consensus is to make treatment decisions for such patients in the same manner as for other incompetent patients.

Physicians should discontinue life-sustaining treatment for patients who have provided advance directives requesting that such treatment be withdrawn. Even without a clear advance directive, the physician and surrogate may ethically decide to withhold life-sustaining treatments through a substituted judgment or an assessment of the patient's best interests. The surrogate may determine that the burdens of continued intervention are disproportionate to any benefits that the patient derives from such treatment. Some physicians believe that there are no medical indications for providing interventions that merely prolong biological existence without any awareness or interaction with the environment. In their view, because patients in a persistent vegetative state cannot experience any benefits or suffer any discomfort, all interventions should be withdrawn. On the other hand, some physicians and families assert that all life is sacred and insist on life-prolonging interventions while accepting that no likelihood of improvement remains. In practice, physicians have shown a tendency to withdraw more complex interventions such as ventilators, renal dialysis, and intensive care from permanently unconscious patients.

INTRAVENOUS FLUIDS AND ARTIFICIAL FEEDINGS

Clinicians disagree about whether to withhold intravenous fluids and tube feedings. The majority position is to regard these as medical interventions with benefits and risks that must be assessed for each patient. Some physicians and families believe, however, that artificial feedings are basic care that may never be withheld or withdrawn and that withholding would constitute discrimination against the vulnerable and disabled. When disagreements occur, physicians must appreciate that opinions on the benefits and burdens of these interventions involve value judgments and religious beliefs, as well as scientific expertise. Physicians with strong beliefs about this matter must follow their conscience in individual cases (*see* "Medicine and the Law"); however, such strong beliefs should be made known to patients or surrogates early in the patient-physician relationship, so patients can seek another physician if they wish. The physician may need to arrange transfer to another physician who is willing to follow the preferences of the patient or surrogate.

Physician-assisted Suicide and Euthanasia

Physician involvement in deliberately hastening a patient's death has long been prohibited in professional codes. The Hippocratic Oath states, "I will give no deadly medicine to anyone if asked, nor suggest any such counsel." Despite ethical and legal prohibitions, some physicians report having provided medications to assist terminally ill patients in ending their lives. When the patient's intent is known to be suicide, the legal risk to physicians who provide specific advice or prescriptions varies by jurisdiction, and the ethics of such actions are in debate. Legal prohibitions against active euthanasia (administration of a lethal agent to end life) exist throughout the Western world, although an open system of tolerance operates in the Netherlands.

Physicians should distinguish among withdrawing life-sustaining treatment, allowing the natural process of death to occur, and taking deliberate actions to shorten a patient's life. Objections to assisted suicide and active euthanasia should not deter physicians from withholding or withdrawing medical interventions in appropriate situations. Indeed, fears that unwanted life-sustaining treatment will be imposed may motivate some patients to request assisted suicide or active euthanasia.

Many physicians feel that physician-assisted suicide and active voluntary euthanasia violate the sanctity of life and compromise their professional role as healers. If euthanasia were to be legalized in a narrow set of circumstances (terminally ill, competent adults who request it), some worry that the application would soon be broadened and abuses would occur (such an unacceptable progression of events is referred to as the "slippery slope") (24). This concern focuses on vulnerable populations, that is, people who are frail, elderly, demented, disabled or very ill and who cannot make their own decisions. By maintaining legal restrictions, the most vulnerable in our society are protected.

Recently, several states considered legalizing euthanasia, raising serious concerns in the medical profession about the ethical aspects of active euthanasia, the role of medicine in society, and the protection of vulnerable populations. We encourage active and thoughtful physician participation in these debates to assure that public policy makers fully consider the needs and vulnerability of patients and the complexity of terminal care.

Some patients who suggest active euthanasia or assisted suicide have untreated depression or uncontrolled pain. The first response of the physician should be to ascertain the concerns and fears of the patient and to check for depression, uncontrolled pain, and other possibly reversible conditions. Patients who are terminally ill and frail, elderly persons are frequently depressed. When the depression is treated, such patients usually no longer wish to die.

Uncontrolled pain may also lead patients to request assisted suicide. Terminally ill patients have inadequate pain control for many reasons. Some uninsured or indigent patients lack access to health care, hospice programs, and other means of adequate pain management. Occasionally, physicians withhold pain medication because they fear that terminally ill patients will become addicted or because they fear medication may hasten death through respiratory suppression. Physicians should make relief of suffering in the terminally ill patient their highest priority (25), as long as this is in accord with the patient's wishes. Ethically, strong support exists for gradually increasing medication in terminal illness to levels that relieve pain, even if a side effect is to shorten life.

The issues are not always clear. In exceptional cases, even optimally administered pain control is inadequate, or the side effects or other symptoms are intolerable. Patients may request pain control and assisted suicide, which directly confronts professional prohibitions. Open conversations between terminally ill patients and their physicians about patient needs and values are essential, even when those conversations include a patient's request for assisted suicide. In most cases, the patient will withdraw the request when pain management, depression, and other concerns have been addressed (26), but occasionally the issue of physician-assisted suicide needs to be explored in depth. However, our society has not yet arrived at a consensus on assisted suicide and most jurisdictions have specific laws prohibiting such action. Physicians and patients must continue to search together for answers to these problems without violating the physician's personal and professional values and without abandoning the patient to struggle alone (27, 28).

The Physician's Relationship to Other Physicians

All physicians share a commitment to care for the sick and to treat each other with integrity and respect in daily professional interactions. The traditional bond between physicians is a powerful aid in the service of patients and must never be used for personal advantage.

Teaching

The very title "doctor," from the Latin *docere*, "to teach," implies that physicians have a responsibility to share knowledge and information with colleagues and with patients. This sharing includes teaching clinical skills and reporting results of scientific research to colleagues, medical students, resident physicians, and other health care providers. It includes communicating clearly with patients and teaching them so that they are properly prepared to participate in their care and in the maintenance of their health.

Physicians in Training

The physician has a responsibility to teach the science, art, and ethics of medicine to medical students, resident physicians, and others and to supervise those in training. In the teaching environment, graded authority for patient management can be delegated to residents, with adequate supervision. It is unethical, however, to delegate authority for patient care to anyone, including another physician, who is not appropriately qualified and experienced. On a teaching service, ultimate responsibility for patient welfare and quality of care remains with the patient's attending physician of record.

Residents often play multiple roles in providing patient care, furthering their own education, and teaching medical students and are bound by the same ethical principles as other physicians. Patients should be made aware of the resident's training status. Residents should acknowledge their limitations and ask for help or supervision from the attending physician, chief of service, or consultants when concerns arise about patient care or the ability of others to perform their duties. Residents must keep the attending physician informed about each patient's hospital course and treatment plans. Residents are not obligated to carry out a treatment plan if it poses major ethical or religious concerns. In such situations, the resident may withdraw from the case after in-depth discussion with the attending physician and after adequate coverage for the patient has been arranged.

Consultation

Physicians should obtain consultation when they feel a need for assistance in caring for the patient or when it is requested by the patient or a legally authorized representative. The level of consultation needed should be established first: a one-visit opinion, continuing cooperative care, or total transfer of authority to the consultant. The consultant should carefully and respectfully explain recommendations to the referring physician and obtain concurrence for major procedures or for additional consultants. The patient, along with the proper records, should be transferred back to the referring physician when the consultation is completed. The referring physician's authority should be respected in this process.

The welfare of the patient is always paramount in the consultation process. Consultants who need temporary charge of the patient's care should obtain the referring physician's cooperation and assent. The referring physician who does not agree with the consultant's recommendations is free to call in another consultant. Differences between the referring physician and the consultant should be resolved based on what is best for the patient (*see* "Peer Review"). The referring physician should receive no fee from the consultant.

A complex clinical situation may call for multiple consultations. One physician must remain in charge of overall care, communicating with the patient and coordinating care based on information derived from the consultations. Unless authority has been formally transferred elsewhere, the ultimate responsibility for the patient's care lies with the referring physician.

The Impaired Physician

Patient care must never be compromised because a physician's judgment or skill is impaired. Physicians significantly impaired for any reason must refrain from activities that may harm patients and should seek assistance in caring for their patients.

Every physician is responsible for protecting patients from an impaired physician and for assisting a colleague whose professional capability is impaired. Physicians are reluctant to identify an impaired colleague, for fear of being wrong, of embarrassment, or of possible litigation.

The identifying physician may find it helpful to discuss the issue with the departmental chair or a senior member of the staff or community. Identification of an impaired colleague should not be delayed, however, because patients may be harmed (29).

A physician's incapacity may result from use of habit-forming agents (alcohol or other substances) or from psychiatric, physiologic, or behavioral disorders. Impairment may also be caused by diseases that affect the cognitive or motor skills necessary to provide adequate care. A physician who feels unable to help an impaired colleague should suggest other sources of help. The legal responsibility of a physician to report such incapacity varies among states, but there is a clear ethical responsibility to report an incapacitated physician to an appropriate authority (such as a chief of service, chief of staff, institutional committee, state medical board, or regulatory agency). Reporting physicians must follow procedures dictated by the hospital, state laws and regulations, and their consciences.

The impaired physician, while undergoing therapy, is entitled to full confidentiality as in any other patient-physician relationship. To protect patients of the impaired physician, someone other than the physician of the impaired physician needs to monitor the impaired physician's fitness to work. Serious conflicts of interest occur if the treating physician tries to fill both roles.

Peer Review

It is unethical for a physician to disparage the professional competence, knowledge, qualifications, or services of another physician to a patient or a third party or to state or imply that a patient has been poorly managed or mistreated by a colleague, without substantial evidence, especially when such behavior is used to recruit patients. Avoiding such inducement is especially necessary for the physician who has been called in as a consultant (*see* "Consultation").

Of equal importance, it is unethical for a physician *not* to report fraud, professional misconduct, incompetence, or abandonment of a patient by another physician. Professional peer review is critical in assuring fair assessment of physician performance for the benefit of the patient. The trust patients and the public invest in physicians requires disclosure to the appropriate authorities and to patients at risk for immediate harm.

All physicians have a duty to participate in peer review. Fear of retaliation, ostracism by colleagues, loss of referrals, or inconvenience is not adequate reason for refusing to participate in peer review. Society looks to physicians to establish professional standards of practice, and this obligation can be met only when all physicians participate in the process. Federal law and most states provide legal protection for physicians who participate in peer review in good faith.

Conversely, in the absence of substantial evidence of professional misconduct, negligence, or incompetence, it is unethical to use the peer review process to exclude another physician from practice, to restrict clinical privileges, or to otherwise harm the physician's practice.

The Physician and Society

Society has conferred professional prerogatives on physicians in the belief that they will use such power for the benefit of patients. In turn, physicians are responsible and accountable to society for their professional actions. Society grants each physician the rights, privileges, and duties pertinent to the patient-physician relationship and has the right to require that physicians be competent and knowledgeable and that they practice with consideration for the patient as a person.

Obligations of the Physician to Society

Physicians have obligations to society that in many ways parallel their obligations to individual patients. Physicians' conduct, both as professionals and as individual citizens, should merit the respect of the community.

All physicians must fulfill the profession's collective responsibility to be advocates for the health of the public. Physicians should protect the public's health by reporting diseases, as required by law, to the responsible authority. They should support public health endeavors that provide the general public with accurate information about health care and comment on medical subjects within their areas of expertise to keep the public properly informed. Physicians should regard interacting with the news media to provide accurate information as an obligation to society and an extension of medical practice.

Physicians should help the community recognize and deal with social and environmental causes of disease. They should work toward ensuring access to health care for all individuals and help correct deficiencies in the availability, accessibility, and quality of health services in the community.

Resource Allocation

Medical care is delivered within social and institutional systems that must take overall resources into account. Increasingly, decisions about resource allocations challenge the physician's traditional role as patient advocate. There have always been limits to this advocacy role; for example, a physician is not obligated to lie to third-party payers for a patient nor to provide all treatments, no matter how futile. Resource allocation pushes these limits further, by asking physicians to consider the best interests of all patients as well as the best interests of each patient. The just allocation of resources presents the physician with ethical dilemmas that cannot be ignored. There is agreement on two fundamental rules:

1. Physicians have a responsibility to use all health-related resources in a technically appropriate and efficient manner. They should plan work-ups carefully and avoid unnecessary testing, medications, operations, and consultations.

2. Decisions on resource allocations must not be made in the context of an individual patient-physician encounter but must be part of a broader social process. Physicians participating in decisions at the policy level should stress the value of health to our society and should base allocations on medical need, cost-effectiveness of treatments, and proper distribution of benefits and burdens in our society.

Relationship of the Physician to Government

The physician should help develop health policy at the local, state, and national levels by expressing views as an individual and as a professional. Through professional activities and associations, as well as through the political process, physicians should participate in health policy decisions. These include societal decisions about the distribution of resources between health care and other social goods and about the various methods for delivering health care, in assuring that no sick person is denied essential medical care.

Physicians must resist being a party to abuses of human rights. Under no circumstances is it ethical for a physician to be used as an instrument of government to do anything to weaken the physical or mental resistance of a human. Neither should a physician participate in, or tolerate, cruel or unusual punishment or disciplinary activities beyond those permitted by the United Nations Standard Minimum Rules for the Treatment of Prisoners (30).

Participation by physicians in the execution of prisoners, except to certify death, is unethical.

Relationship of Physicians to Other Health Professionals

The interests of the patient have primacy in all aspects of the patient-physician relationship. The attending physician should act as an advocate and coordinator of care for the patient and should assume appropriate responsibility, especially when other health professionals help. The physician should collaborate only with competent health professionals when sharing the care of a patient.

All health professionals share a commitment to work together to serve the patient's interests. The best patient care is often a team effort, and mutual respect, cooperation, and communication should govern this effort. Even though health professionals have special areas of expertise, each member of the patient care team has equal moral status. When a health professional has major ethical objections to an attending physician's order, both should discuss the matter thoroughly. Mechanisms should be available in hospitals to resolve differences of opinion among members of the patient care team.

Ethics Committees and Ethics Consultants

Ethics committees and consultants contribute to achieving patient care goals primarily by developing educational programs in the institution, coordinating institutional resources, providing a forum for discussion among medical and hospital professionals, and assisting institutions to develop sound policies and practices. Although it is generally agreed that neither ethics committees nor consultants should have decision making authority, they can advise physicians on ethical matters.

Medicine and the Law

Physicians should remember that all citizens are equal under the law, and being ill does not diminish the right or expectation to be treated equally. Stated another way, illness does not, in and of itself, change a patient's legal rights or permit a physician to ignore those legal rights.

The law is society's mechanism for establishing boundaries for conduct. Society has a right to expect that those boundaries will not be disregarded. In instances of conflict, the physician must decide whether to violate the law for the sake of what he or she considers to be the dictates of medical ethics. Such a violation may jeopardize the physician's legal position or the legal rights of the patient. It should be remembered that ethical concepts are not always fully reflected in or adopted by the law. Violation of the law for purposes of complying with one's ethical standards may have significant consequences for the physician and should only be undertaken after thorough consideration and, generally, after obtaining legal counsel.

EXPERT WITNESSES

Physicians have specialized knowledge and expertise that may be needed in judicial or administrative processes. Often, expert testimony is necessary for a court or administrative agency to understand the patient's condition, treatment, and prognosis. Physicians may be reluctant to become involved in legal proceedings because the process is unfamiliar and time-consuming. Their absence may mean, however, that legal decisions are made without the benefit of all medical facts or opinions. Without the participation of physicians, the mechanisms used to resolve many disputes, and patients themselves, may suffer.

Although physicians cannot be compelled to participate as expert witnesses, the profession as a whole has the ethical duty to assist patients and society in resolving disputes (31). In this role, physicians must give an honest and objective interpretation and representation of the medical facts. Physicians are entitled to reasonable compensation for the time and expenses incurred as expert witnesses.

Strikes by Physicians

It is unethical for physicians to withhold medical services through strikes when patients will be harmed or when the strike is for physicians' benefit. Physicians individually and as a group have sufficient social position, political awareness, and initiative to find other methods to deal with problems that justify drastic social and political action and are obligated to exhaust all alternatives to strikes.

Research

Medical progress and improved patient care depend on innovative and vigorous research. The basic principle of research is honesty, which must be assured by institutional protocols. Fraud in research must be condemned and punished. Honesty and integrity must govern all stages of research, from the initial grant application to publication of results. Reviewers of grant applications and journal articles must respect the confidentiality of new ideas and information; they must not use what they learn from the review process for their own purposes, nor should they misrepresent ideas of others as their own.

Scientists have a responsibility to provide research results of high quality; to gather data meticulously; to keep impeccable records of work done; to interpret results objectively, not forcing them into preconceived molds or models; to submit their work to peer review; and to report new knowledge. Self-aggrandizement, public acclaim, recognition by professional peers, or financial gain should never be primary motivations in scientific research.

Authors of research reports must be well enough acquainted with the work being reported that they can take public responsibility for the integrity of the study and the validity of the findings, and they must have substantially contributed to the research itself. Sources of funding for the research project must be disclosed to potential collaborators in the research and listed in publications (*see* "Conflicts of Interest").

Advances in medical knowledge and technology sometimes occur rapidly. The clinical application of such progress occurs before the medical community has had an opportunity to establish guidelines for appropriate and ethical use. The medical profession is responsible for ensuring verification of the safety and efficacy of new technologies and treatment. Medical consensus development should be open to public scrutiny.

Clinical Investigation

Advances in the diagnosis and treatment of disease are based on well-designed, carefully controlled, and ethically conducted clinical studies. The medical profession must assume the responsibility for assuring that the research is worth doing. Subjects must be equitably selected and instructed concerning the nature of the research; consent from the subject or an authorized representative (32) must be truly informed and given freely; research must be planned thoughtfully, so that it has a high probability of yielding significant results; risks to patients must be minimized; and the benefit/risk ratio must be sufficiently high to justify the research effort.

Each institution receiving federal support for research on human subjects is required to create an institutional review board. All proposed clinical research, regardless of the source of support, should be approved by the local institutional review board to assure that the research plans are reasonable and that research subjects are adequately protected.

Although this formal system of review is designed to protect research subjects, the premise on which all ethical research is based is mutual trust and respect between research subjects and researchers. This premise requires that physician-investigators involved in designing or carrying out research have primary concern for the potential subjects of these investigations.

Although the responsibility for assuring reasonable protection of human subjects resides with the investigators and the local institutional review board, the medical profession as a whole also has responsibilities. Physicians referring patients for participation in research protocols must satisfy themselves that the program follows established ethical guidelines and provides for realistic informed consent, reasonable assurances of safety, and an acceptable benefit/risk ratio. If the research risks become too great or if continued participation cannot be justified, the physician must be willing to advise the patient to withdraw. Physicians-of-record should not abdicate overall responsibility for patients they have referred to a research project. Giving finder's fees to individual physicians for referring patients to a research project raises the issue of conflict of interest and is unethical.

Innovative Medical Therapies

The use of innovative medical therapies falls along the continuum between established practice and research. Innovative therapies include the use of unconventional dosages of standard medications, previously untried applications of known procedures, and the use of approved drugs for nonapproved indications. The primary purpose of innovative medical therapies is to benefit the individual patient. Clinicians will confront the ethical dilemmas of innovative practice more frequently than the ethical problems concerning medical research. Important medical advances have emerged from successful innovations, but innovation should always be approached carefully. When there is no precedent for an innovative therapy, consultation with peers, an institutional review board, or other expert group is necessary to assess whether the innovation is in the patient's best interest, the risks of the innovation, and probable outcomes of not using a standard therapy (33). Informed consent is particularly important; patients need to understand that the therapy is not standard treatment (34).

Scientific Publication

Scientists build on the published work of other researchers. As stated earlier, scientists can proceed with confidence only if they can assume that the previously reported facts on which their work is based have been reported accurately. All scientists have a professional responsibility to be honest in their publications: describing methods accurately and in sufficient detail; reporting only observations that were actually made; making clear in the manuscript what information derives from the author's work and what comes from others (and where it was published); assuring readers that research has been carried out in accordance with ethical principles; and assigning authorship only to persons meriting and accepting authorship (35).

Plagiarism is unethical. Incorporating the words of others or one's own published words, either verbatim or by paraphrasing without appropriate attribution, is unethical and may have legal consequences.

Public Announcement of Research Discoveries

In this era of rapid communication and intense media and public interest in medical news, it has become common for clinical investigators or their institutions to call press conferences and make public announcements of new research developments. Although it is desirable for the media to obtain accurate information about scientific developments, researchers should approach public pronouncements carefully, using language that does not invite misinterpretation or unjustified extrapolation.

Generally, press releases should be issued and press conferences held only after the research has been published in a peer-reviewed journal, so that the details of the study are available to the scientific community. Statements of scientists receive great visibility. An "announcement of preliminary results," even couched in the most careful terms, is frequently reported by the media as a "breakthrough." Care must be taken to avoid raising false public expectations and embarrassing the scientists involved, which reduce the credibility of the scientific community as a whole.

Conclusion

We hope this manual will help physicians, whether clinicians or research scientists, address some of the challenging ethical dilemmas that confront us each day. The manual is written by physicians for physicians, as we all attempt to find our way through difficult terrain. The ultimate intent of any medical ethics guideline, however, is to improve the quality of care provided to patients.

Acknowledgments: The American College of Physicians and the ACP Ethics Committee are solely responsible for the contents of the *Manual*. Both, however, would like to recognize former Ethics Committee members who made significant contributions to the development of this manual through their reviews of drafts: Jeremiah A. Barondess, MD; Michael Bernstein, MD; John F. Burnum, MD; Harriet P. Dustan, MD; Saul J. Farber, MD; Norton J. Greenberger, MD; Eugene A. Hildreth, MD; Richard J. Kahn, MD; C. S. Lewis, Jr., MD; Robert H. Moser, MD; E. D. Pellegrino, MD; Richard J. Reitemeier, MD; Richard W. Vilter, MD; Ralph O. Wallerstein, MD; and Donald E. Wilson, MD.

We would also like to express much gratitude to other reviewers of the *Manual*: Patricia P. Barry, MD, MPH; James J. Bergin, MD; Richard W. Besdine, MD; James L. Borland, Jr., MD; Dan W. Brock, PhD; Nadine C. Bruce, MD; Arthur L. Caplan, PhD; Christine K. Cassel, MD; Clifton R. Cleaveland, MD; Linda Hawes Clever, MD; Frank Davidoff, MD; L. L. Emanuel, MD, PhD; H. Tristam Engelhardt, Jr., PhD, MD; Robert L. Fine, MD; Harold M. Friedman, MD; Michael A. Grodin, MD; Abraham L. Halpern, MD; Frederick F. Holmes, MD; Edward J. Huth, MD; Albert R. Jonsen, PhD; A. Martin Lerner, MD; Robert J. Levine, MD; Joanne Lynn, MD, MA; John P. Mullooly, MD; Lynn Peterson, MD; Timothy

E. Quill, MD; James D. Rogge, MD; Laurence Z. Rubenstein, MD; Charles G. Sasser, MD; Alan M. Siegal, MD; George G. Spellman, Sr., MD; Norton Spritz, MD, JD; Sara Ellen Walker, MD; James Webster, MS, MD; Mark E. Williams, MD; and Stuart J. Youngner, MD.

References

1. **American College of Physicians.** American College of Physicians Ethics Manual. Second edition. Ann Intern Med. 1989;111:245-52, 317-35.
2. **Jonsen AR.** The New Medicine and the Old Ethics. Cambridge, Massachusetts: Harvard University Press; 1990.
3. **Reiser SJ, Dyck AJ, Curran WJ.** Ethics in Medicine: Historical Perspectives and Contemporary Concerns. Cambridge, Massachusetts: MIT Press; 1977.
4. **Rothman DJ.** Strangers at the Bedside: A History of How Law and Bioethics Transformed Medical Decision Making. New York: Basic Books; 1991.
5. **Veatch RM.** A Theory of Medical Ethics. New York: Basic Books; 1981.
6. **Beauchamp TL, Childress JR.** Principles of Biomedical Ethics. Third edition. New York: Oxford University Press, 1989.
7. **President's Commission for the Study of Ethical Problems in Medicine and Biomedical and Behavioral Research.** Making Health Care Decisions: A Report on the Ethical and Legal Implications of Informed Consent in the Patient-Practitioner Relationship. Washington, DC: U.S. Government Printing Office; 1982.
8. **Katz J.** The Silent World of Doctor and Patient. New York: The Free Press; 1984.
9. **President's Commission for the Study of Ethical Problems in Medicine and Biomedical and Behavioral Research.** Securing Access to Health Care: A Report on the Ethical Implications of Differences in the Availability of Health Services. Washington, DC: U.S. Government Printing Office; 1983.
10. **President's Commission for the Study of Ethical Problems in Medicine and Biomedical and Behavioral Research.** Screening and Counseling for Genetic Conditions: A Report on the Ethical, Social, and Legal Implications of Genetic Screening, Counseling, and Educational Programs. Washington, DC: U.S. Government Printing Office; 1983.
11. **President's Commission for the Study of Ethical Problems in Medicine and Biomedical and Behavioral Research.** Splicing Life: A Report on the Social and Ethical Issues of Genetic Engineering with Human Beings. Washington, DC: U.S. Government Printing Office; 1982.
12. **President's Commission for the Study of Ethical Problems in Medicine and Biomedical and Behavioral Research.** Deciding to Forego Life-sustaining Treatment: A Report on the Ethical, Medical, and Legal Issues in Treatment Decisions. Washington, DC: U.S. Government Printing Office; 1983.
13. **The Hastings Center.** Guidelines on the Termination of Life-sustaining Treatment and the Care of the Dying. Briarcliff Manor, New York: The Hastings Center; 1987.
14. **American College of Physicians.** Health care needs of the adolescent. Ann Intern Med. 1989;110:930-5.
15. **Burnum JF.** Secrets about patients. N Engl J Med. 1991;324:1130-3.

16. **American College of Physicians.** Ethics case study: defining the duty to treat HIV-positive patients. ACP Observer. 1991;11:1,5,8.
17. **American College of Physicians and the Infectious Diseases Society of America.** The acquired immunodeficiency syndrome (AIDS) and infection with the human immunodeficiency virus (HIV). Ann Intern Med. 1988;108:460-9.
18. **La Puma J, Stocking CB, La Voie D, Darling CA.** When physicians treat members of their own families. Practice in a community hospital. N Engl J Med.1991;325:1290-4.
19. **American Medical Association, Council on Ethical and Judicial Affairs.** Sexual misconduct in the practice of medicine. JAMA. 1991;266:2741-5.
20. **American College of Physicians.** Ethics case study: when finances may influence physician decision-making. ACP Observer. 1990;10:1,8,9,12.
21. **American Medical Association, Council on Ethical and Judicial Affairs.** Current Opinions of the Council of Ethical and Judicial Affairs of the American Medical Association. AMA Council Report C/I-91: 6,7.
22. **American College of Physicians.** Physicians and the pharmaceutical industry. Ann Intern Med. 1990;112:624-6.
23. The relationship between physicians and the pharmaceutical industry. A report of the Royal College of Physicians. J R Coll Physicians Lond. 1986;20:235-42.
24. **Brock DW.** Voluntary active euthanasia. Hastings Cent Rep. 1992;22:10-22.
25. Acute Pain Management in Adults: Operative Procedures. Quick Reference Guide for Clinicians. AHCPR Pub. No. 92-0019. Rockville, Maryland: Agency for Health Care Policy and Research, Public Health Service, U.S. Department of Health and Human Services.
26. **van Der Maas PJ, van Delden JJ, Pijnenborg L, Looman CW.** Euthanasia and other medical decisions concerning the end of life. Lancet.1991; 338:669-74.
27. **Blendon RJ, Szalay US, Knox RA.** Should physicians aid their patients in dying? The public perspective. JAMA. 1992; 267:2658-62.
28. **American College of Physicians.** Ethics case study: Ms. Washington is terminally ill and wants to die. Should Dr. Jones assist? ACP Observer. 1991;10:1,20,21.
29. **American College of Physicians.** Ethics case study: the dilemma of dealing with an impaired colleague. ACP Observer. 1991;11: 10,11.
30. **United Nations, First Congress on the Prevention of Crime and the Treatment of Offenders.** Standard Minimum Rules for the Treatment of Prisoners; 1955.
31. **American College of Physicians.** Guidelines for the physician expert witness. Ann Intern Med. 1990;113:789.
32. **American College of Physicians.** Cognitively impaired subjects. Ann Intern Med. 1989; 111:843-8.
33. **Lind SE.** Innovative medical therapies: between practice and research. Clin Res. 1988; 36: 546-51.
34. **Levine RJ.** Ethics and Regulation of Clinical Research. Baltimore: Urban & Schwarzenberg; 1986.
35. **International Committee of Medical Journal Editors.** Uniform requirements for manuscripts submitted to biomedical journals. N Engl J Med. 1991;324:424-8.

Ethics Case Study: When Finances May Influence Physician Decision-Making

This is the first in an occasional series of case studies on ethics with commentaries developed by the College's Ethics Committee. This series will elaborate on controversial and subtle aspects of issues not previously addressed in detail in the ACP Ethics Manual *or other College position statements, and to make our policies more relevant to daily practice by discussing their application in specific situations. The most relevant issues and concerns of all, however, are those that are identified by our members.*

We hope this series will prove valuable.

Edwin P. Maynard, MD, MACP
Chair, ACP Ethics Committee

The following case history presents an example of the potential influence of financial incentives on physicians' clinical decision-making. A common medical scenario is presented in which there is potential influence from the organizational setting and the contractual arrangements under which the care is provided.

Case History

Ted and Ned are 46-year-old, asymptomatic, sedentary identical twins. Both are executives in local corporations. Former smokers—both smoked about one-half pack per day from their late teens to their early 30s, when they quit as a New Year's resolution—they have been generally healthy except for mild obesity, secondary to many executive lunches. As a New Year's resolution for 1990, Ted and Ned agree to join a local gym to "tone up" and get back in shape (both had been college athletes). The gym required a note from the men's doctors before they could start the exercise program, but no specific tests were mandated.

Ted had enrolled in GreatCare, an IPA-model HMO, because he liked the "comprehensive care" concept, including an emphasis on prevention and wellness. He also valued the idea of no out-of-pocket health care costs other than the premium deducted from his paycheck. Because it is an IPA-model HMO, in which the HMO contracts with independent providers in private practice, Ted was able to select a local physician about whom he had heard good things.

Unbeknownst to Ted, his physician had agreed to certain contractual arrangements with the HMO. Among them were a 15% discount in his usual fees and an additional 15% withholding. The HMO would return the 15% withholding to the physician only if his referral account for specialist services and laboratory tests had a surplus at the end of the year. If the referral account had a surplus, the physician would get his withheld funds and a bonus equal to half of his share of any surplus in the referral pool. The HMO, which had grouped Ted's physician with four others in his community as a risk pool, provided him with the names, addresses and telephone numbers of these other physicians and encouraged him to contact the group to "discuss the use of referral funds from their aggregate pool."

Ned had elected traditional indemnity fee-for-service health care insurance, in which his premiums and out-of-pocket payments were higher than Ted's. He felt that it was important to retain complete freedom of choice with respect to doctors, despite the somewhat higher overall costs. As is usual in traditional fee-for-service health care, Ned's doctor is paid for each patient visit and every service performed.

Ted and Ned met at the gym for their first joint workout. Ned explained that his physician would not write a note for him to start the program without first performing an ECG and exercise tolerance test (results of both were normal). Ned takes some pride in what he considers to be his doctor's comprehensive approach to his health care, and the extra attention he got for clearance for the exercise program. Ted wants to know why his doctor hadn't ordered the tests also. After some thought, Ned begins to wonder if the expensive and time-consuming tests he received really were needed. Both brothers are confused.

Commentary

The physician's primary obligations are to the patient, not to the system under which he provides care, and certainly not to the physician's own pocketbook. It is obviously easiest to follow the ethical course under medically clear circumstances: An exercise tolerance test would be medically unnecessary for a 20-year-old female college athlete, about to join a gym, who has no risk factors.

Many situations require physician judgment as to whether an intervention or test is appropriate given the individual patient. The objectivity of physician discretion must not be allowed to be affected by external forces.

Says the *ACP Ethics Manual*: "The welfare of the patient must at all times be paramount, and the physician must insist that the medically appropriate level of care takes primacy over fiscal considerations. . . . The guiding principle should always be care consistent with humanistic, scientific and efficient medicine. . . . In the final analysis, no external factors should interfere with the dedication of the physician to provide optimal care for his or her patient" (1).

In addition to obvious influences on behavior, physicians must be aware of more subtle influences that could affect judgment when the best clinical decision for an individual patient is unclear; for example, in the fee-for-service setting a physician may too quickly recommend a test or procedure, while the HMO physician may adopt a wait-and-see approach for too long (2).

The patient-physician relationship necessarily involves unequal partners. Vulnerable patients entrust their health and lives to physicians, the keepers and communicators of medical knowledge. Patients have the right to make informed decisions about their care. But physicians have the power to influence decision-making.

With fee-for-service, more tests mean more fees. Physicians must be aware of, and seek to avoid, the "more is better" philosophy that this setting might implicitly encourage. Some commentators have said that potential conflict is easier for the patient to see in this setting; patients know that the more the doctor does, the more patients (or insurers) pay. The patient's ability to verify the medical need for a service by getting a second opinion can serve as a check on physician behavior (3).

That certainly holds true regarding the need for a major operation, but Ned has no reason to question his doctor's judgment that exercise testing is required in order to evaluate whether he can join the gym. And even if the second opinion "check" theory were applicable more often, it would not convert behavior that was ethically unacceptable into ethically acceptable behavior.

In the HMO setting, if a medically needed service is denied because incentives distort physician judgment, rather than merely encourage cost-effective care, the patient may be unlikely to know it. Here, there has been no discourse between physician and patient. In the fee-for-service context something affirmative has to happen before the physician profits—the physician must *propose* the service and perform the test. If the physician refers the patient elsewhere, and if something other than appropriate care motivates the referral, it raises issues ranging from fee-splitting to unnecessary referrals.

In the HMO setting, the patient may not know a type of care is being *omitted*. Some patients may question what they see as a lack of care, if they expected to undergo a test or receive a prescription, for example, but others may not know what care may be missing.

A number of lawsuits naming HMOs as defendants are now making their way through the courts. Plaintiffs have alleged that HMO incentive systems, which had not been disclosed to them, compromised the independent judgment of primary physicians, resulting in poor health care services. Physicians can themselves end up as defendants. In the fee-for-service setting, fear of lawsuits has been cited as the basis for so-called "defensive medicine," but this does not justify providing unnecessary care. The practice and documentation of medically appropriate care remain the best defense in a medical malpractice action. The threat of lawsuits should no more affect care than clinical judgment should be distorted by financial incentives.

In a fee-for-service practice, a physician may consciously or unconsciously over-test. In using tests appropriately, physicians must look not only at the immediate costs of a test, but consider that additional expenses can mount in the follow-up of an abnormal result that turns out to be a false-positive. Also important are the potential medical complications in the performance of the original test or follow-up, and the anxiety patients may suffer while waiting to find out if they actually have the disease or condition. These are reasons that ACP and others have been developing guidelines for the use of common tests in screening, case-finding, diagnosis and management of disease.

However, a physician attempting to care for Ted or Ned according to ACP's medical necessity guidelines on

"Screening for Asymptomatic Coronary Artery Disease: Exercise Stress Testing" (American College of Physicians, February 1990) and on "Screening for Asymptomatic CAD: The Resting Electrocardiogram" (American College of Physicians, April 1990) would be in a gray zone, and would have to rely on individual judgment.

The exercise stress testing guidelines state:

> Exercise testing is not recommended as a routine screening procedure in adults with no evidence of coronary heart disease and no risk factors. . . . Some asymptomatic persons may have particular reasons to consider exercise stress testing for coronary artery disease. Some persons are especially likely to have the disease because of increased age, male gender and at least one other risk factor (family history of CAD, cigarette smoking, diabetes mellitus, systolic blood pressure greater than 140 mm Hg, hypercholesterolemia, or a cholesterol to HDL ratio of more than 6.0). Other persons who should be tested are those who have an occupation that puts others at risk (for example, bus drivers or airline pilots) or are sedentary and about to begin a program of physical conditioning. There is insufficient evidence to make a strong recommendation for or against use of routine stress testing in these groups.

Similarly, the resting electrocardiogram guidelines list the above risk factors for CAD, and state that: The resting ECG is not recommended as a routine practice in people who are under age 65 and do not have evidence for cardiovascular disease or its risk factors. However, it may be appropriate in selected patients, especially in situations where the published evidence is not decisive.

The fact that the brothers are former cigarette smokers could put them at increased risk for coronary artery disease, but this is not as clear-cut as it would be for current smokers, or those who smoked several packs per day or quit more recently. The fact that each patient is sedentary and mildly obese, and the nature of the exercise program each is about to start, are additional considerations for the physicians to evaluate. Decision-making is also affected by variation in the information elicited by different physicians in the history and physical examination. Styles of diagnosis and management, personalities and the patients' needs and preferences all can affect medical choices.

As long as these and other medical factors were the reasons for the decisions regarding testing, then the best interest of each patient is motivating each physician. As it turns out, each doctors' income was enhanced here because the fee-for-service physician performed the tests on Ned, while the HMO doctor, whose take-home pay could be reduced had he ordered the tests, did not order them for Ted.

Finally, the comparison of the care they received has left both Ned and Ted somewhat confused. Patients need to be able to have confidence in the care they receive, and must always be fully informed about the medical care that they accept. Given the circumstances, Ted's physician probably need not have explained why he was *not* doing tests he felt were not medically indicated (unless the patient had asked about it specifically), though he should explain his reasoning fully when and if Ted raises this at his next visit. Likewise, Ned's physician may need to go into greater detail at Ned's request. Decisions that patients *perceive* as conflicts of interest on the part of their physicians can undermine the patient-physician relationship.

Conclusion

Physicians have an ethical duty to be aware of the financial incentives of the system in which they practice and the possibility of obvious and subtle influences. Disclosing financial incentives and interests might provide patients with needed information, although this is not necessarily a remedy to conflicts. Little has been written about the mechanics of disclosure such as how and what information should be presented and oversight measures to ensure compliance (4).

Disclosure might range from physician statements about ownership interests in a laboratory or other health care entity to which the physician refers patients, to explanations of the incentives of particular practice settings. Physicians are not relieved of their obligation to serve the best interests of their patients, however, whether or not they, or the corporate bodies for which they work, disclose the relevant financial incentives under which they practice medicine.

Acknowledgments: The Ethics Committee would like to thank Alan L. Hillman, MD, MBA, FACP, and Lois Snyder, JD, ACP's Manager of Health and Medical-Legal Policy Development, primary authors of this first case history and commentary, respectively.

References

1. **American College of Physicians**. American College of Physicians Ethics Manual. Part 1: History; The Patient; Other Physicians. Ann Intern Med. 1989; 111: 245-52; Part 2: The Physician and Society; Research: Life-Sustaining Treatment; Other Issues. Ann Intern Med. 1989; 111: 327-35.
2. **Hillman A**. Health maintenance organizations, financial incentives and physicians' judgments. Ann Intern Med. 1990; 112: 891-3.
3. **Morreim H**. Conflicts of interest: Profits and problems in physician referrals. JAMA. 1989; 262: 390-4.
4. **Rodwin M**. Physicians' conflicts of interest: The limitations of disclosure. N Engl J Med. 1989; 321: 1405-8.

Ethics Case Study: Defining the Duty to Treat HIV-Positive Patients

Case History

John Alden, 40, has chronic, stable angina that does not respond to medical therapies. He returns to Dr. Standish, an internist who has followed him for five years. In taking the interval history, Dr. Standish finds that Mr. Alden had HIV testing a year ago at an anonymous site and is HIV-positive. Mr. Alden reports that he feels well in general, but has noticed significant worsening of his chest pain. His physical examination is unchanged. Because of the change in Mr. Alden's cardiac symptoms, Dr. Standish orders an exercise thallium scan, which suggests two-vessel involvement.

Dr. Standish has privileges at Sheridan Hospital. He refers Mr. Alden to Dr. Montgomery, head of cardiology there, for a same-day catheterization. Dr. Montgomery, in reviewing the medical records, notes that Mr. Alden is HIV-positive. He states that he and his staff have decided to refuse to perform elective cardiac caths on HIV-positive patients. Dr. Standish accuses Dr. Montgomery of gross dereliction of his duty to patients.

Dr. Montgomery is offended. He claims the risk of HIV transmission to his staff far outweighs the benefits for the patient, especially in the long term. He explains that this decision was not made lightly; it was in response to the recent discovery that his chief resident seroconverted after exposure to the virus during a procedure. Subsequently, the entire medical staff petitioned the hospital to test all patients for HIV on admission; the request was denied because of legal concerns and inadequate counseling services for HIV-positive patients.

The medical staff strongly believes that universal precautions do not adequately protect physicians doing invasive procedures. Also, the housestaff has no life or disability insurance in the event of HIV infection. Because the hospital is in an area of high HIV prevalence, the staff deemed these risks unacceptably high. Dr. Montgomery says that the hospital administration, while not fully agreeing with this position, supports the staff's decision. He believes Mr. Alden's best interests would be served by referring him to another cardiac care center.

Dr. Standish is sympathetic, but remains unpersuaded. He will not be able to follow Mr. Alden through his cath, possible surgery and recovery at another hospital. He wonders what to say to Mr. Alden, and what this experience tells him about voluntary HIV testing.

Commentary

The College, among other groups, has upheld the physician's "duty to treat" AIDS and HIV-positive patients, drawing upon the professionalism of medicine. "It is inappropriate for any health care professional to compromise the treatment of any patient, including those with transmissible, lethal diseases such as AIDS, on the grounds that such patients present unacceptable medical risks" (1). The *ACP Ethics Manual* states that "a physician may not discriminate against a class or category of patients. . . ." (2). This case study illustrates the difficulties and conflicts physicians may face in fulfilling their obligations to patients. In practical terms, no obligation is absolute. What are the boundaries of this duty to treat, and how can ethical parameters guide individual physicians in the wake of AIDS?

The ethical imperative to treat AIDS patients stems from the duty to treat all classes of patients within a physician's sphere of competence. While a physician is not obligated to treat any one patient (except in certain circumstances, such as in an emergency room or on call), refusing to treat entire groups of people violates the values of professional responsibility.

Contrast this with a more commercial model of physician responsibility, in which physicians are not obligated to treat any person or group. In this model, medicine is more like a trade; physicians are business people who sell their skills to consumers (patients), and become obligated only through contractual arrangements (3).

The College has consistently rejected this as the sole interpretation of the physician-patient relationship. "The practice of medicine is a societal trust and carries with it a societal responsibility. If medicine wishes to retain its respected status as the healing profession, we must continue to provide the best possible care to our patients, regardless of risk" (1).

Assuming that the physicians in this example accept this notion of professional responsibility, how can we understand their different positions? Dr. Standish wants to provide the best care he can to Mr. Alden by referring him appropriately and following him through the length of his hospital stay and recovery. He believes that Mr. Alden's HIV status does not preclude an elective workup of angina, since the patient is asymptomatic (for HIV infection) and he is likely to live many years. As a general internist, Dr. Standish does not do invasive procedures and believes universal precautions adequately protect him from HIV infection.

Dr. Montgomery, on the other hand, runs the cardiac cath lab, where parenteral blood exposures occur frequently. One staff member has already seroconverted, and Dr. Montgomery has heard estimates of a 0.5% to 12% annual risk of infection for surgeons and other physicians doing invasive procedures in high prevalence areas (4, 5). He believes the cumulative risk of death is unacceptable for his staff, especially when weighed against the marginal benefits to many HIV-positive patients.

But recent data do not support the magnitude of risk that Dr. Montgomery presupposes. The cumulative risk for HIV infection in health care workers depends on three variables: the prevalence of the virus in the patient population; the frequency of needlestick exposures; and the risk of seroconversion from a single contaminated needlestick (5). In a study of surgical personnel at the San Francisco General Hospital, Gerberding and colleagues calculate a theoretical risk for occupational HIV infection of 0.125 infections per year, or one infection among surgical personnel every eight years (6). As the authors state, even this level of risk represents a major life-threatening occupational hazard for surgical personnel at San Francisco General. In places of average (less than 3%) HIV prevalence, the risk would be reduced to one infection in the surgical staff every 80 years.

Dr. Montgomery also confuses the equation in medical decision-making by weighing the risks to the physician against the benefits to the patient. Clinical indications consist of the *patient's* risks and benefits; while an elective cardiac workup may not be indicated for an acutely ill

AIDS patient, that decision is based on medical futility (itself a complex, controversial issue). Dr. Montgomery would have to prove that the prognosis *for Mr. Alden* makes the workup futile—an untenable position these days.

Nevertheless, Dr. Montgomery does have a moral responsibility to minimize the risk to his staff. He is on more solid ethical footing if the results of routine HIV testing are used to manage risk without compromising patient care. This is true only if evidence indicates physician knowledge of the patient's HIV status reduces risk to the medical staff, and if all patients give truly informed consent. There is some evidence against the first point; in fact, some commentators have suggested that HIV testing of patients will put physicians at *greater* risk because they will be reassured by negative results, some of which will be false.

Lastly, Dr. Montgomery believes that the current climate of fear and hesitation at Sheridan Hospital, given the chief resident's seroconversion, precludes providing optimal care to Mr. Alden. Since there are a number of other cardiac care centers nearby, he does not feel that he has abrogated his professional responsibility to patients, and has achieved a delicate balance between his "duty to treat" and his moral obligation to his staff.

Dr. Standish cannot agree. While he acknowledges that Mr. Alden can get good care at another hospital, he does not believe that the staff at Sheridan Hospital has fulfilled its duties. He recognizes that referring his patient elsewhere may be the best compromise in this instance. But his patient may suffer from the discontinuity of care and spend more time and money traveling to another center. Dr. Standish is also concerned about the staff's categorical refusal to treat HIV-positive patients. How can medicine, as a profession, meet its collective obligation to patients if all physicians do not share the burden?

The "duty to treat" has little meaning if fear or inexperience excuses physicians from their responsibilities. It is disingenuous, and somewhat circular, for a physician to claim that fear of a class of patients precludes optimal care and justifies refusing to treat the entire class. Fear and deliberate inexperience can interfere with patient care, but physicians have a moral responsibility to confront and overcome personal barriers, rather than just referring patients to other physicians.

In turn, medical institutions have a responsibility to minimize the actual and perceived risk to their medical staffs. As one HIV-positive resident wrote, "A safe work environment also means one in which health workers are well protected economically, with appropriate health, disability and life insurance" (7). Sheridan Hospital might arrange lectures and discussions about HIV and its transmission; train the staff in universal precautions and stress strict adherence to them; invite the staff to suggest further precautions that might enhance safety without compromising patient care; and review life and disability coverage to ensure adequate financial protection for the entire staff.

Finally, after confronting fear and overcoming inexperience, physicians must grapple with the bounds of acceptable risk. Some risks are too great even for dedicated professionals. Soldiers are not duty-bound to perform suicide missions, nor are firefighters required to enter buildings on the verge of collapse (5). The occupational risk of HIV transmission should be judged relative to risks faced by other professionals, and to other risks faced by physicians.

Conflicts surrounding hazardous duty have existed as long as the medical profession itself; history reveals that physicians struggled with ethical conduct in the face of epidemics such as bubonic plague, yellow fever, smallpox and cholera, often surrounded by large and largely uninvestigated risks to their lives (8). Some physicians fled or refused to treat the victims; others cared selflessly for all the sick and some died with their patients.

So while occupational risk is not new to physicians, AIDS has introduced the problem to generations of physicians relatively unaccustomed to confronting real personal danger as they deliver medical care. The stigma of the diagnosis, the devastation of the illness itself and persistent media attention have combined to highlight this occupational risk above all others.

In fact, physicians are at far greater risk for hepatitis B and tuberculosis infection than HIV infection. An estimated 12,000 health care workers become infected yearly with the hepatitis B virus (HBV), and 250 eventually die from it (9). Of all health care workers, 15%-30% show evidence of exposure to HBV, which is far more infectious than HIV. The risk of HIV infection after needlestick exposure to contaminated blood is 0.5%, compared with

6%-30% for HBV. Despite the availability of a fairly effective vaccine, many physicians do not protect themselves against HBV infection (10). Clearly, physicians accept this level of occupational risk, and refusing to treat HIV-positive patients must be viewed in this context. AIDS has provoked a degree of fear unparalleled in recent memory, a fear to which physicians are not immune.

In a recent national survey (11), 75% of 2,450 physician respondents agreed with the following statement: "A physician may not ethically refuse to treat a patient whose condition is within the physician's current realm of competence solely because the patient is seropositive (for HIV)." However, there were statistically significant differences among and within specialties. General internists (85%) were more likely than internal medicine subspecialists (73%) to agree with the statement. While the precise reasons for this pattern are unclear, the authors noted that many medical subspecialists perform procedures that may increase their perceived risk. General surgeons (69%), surgical specialists (59%) and obstetricians/gynecologists (64%) were less likely to feel that physicians have an ethical responsibility to treat HIV-positive patients.

AIDS offers us a critical test of the ethical parameters of the duty to treat, as well as an opportunity to reaffirm medical values and principles. By societal and professional standards, the College reaffirms the ethical imperative to deliver quality care to HIV-positive and AIDS patients.

Acknowledgments: The committee would like to thank Janet Weiner, MPH, primary author of this case history and commentary.

References

1. **Health and Public Policy Committee, American College of Physicians and the Infectious Disease Society of America.** The acquired immunodeficiency syndrome (AIDS) and infection with the human immunodeficiency virus (HIV). Ann Intern Med. 1988; 108:460-9.
2. **Ethics Committee, American College of Physicians.** American College of Physicians Ethics Manual, Part 1. Ann Intern Med. 1989; 111:245-52.
3. **Annas GJ**. Not saints, but healers: The legal duties of health care professionals in the AIDS epidemic. Am J Pub Health. 1988; 78:844-9.
4. **Task Force on AIDS and Orthopedic Surgery**. Recommendations for the Prevention of Human Immunodeficiency Virus (HIV) Transmission in the Practice of Orthopedic Surgery. American Academy of Orthopedic Surgeons, July 1989.

5. **Emanuel EJ**. Do physicians have an obligation to treat patients with AIDS? N Engl J Med. 1988; 318:1686-90.
6. **Gerberding JL, Littell C, Tarkington A, Brown A, Schecter WP**. Risk of exposure of surgical personnel to patients' blood during surgery at San Francisco General Hospital. N Engl J Med. 1990; 322:1788-93.
7. **Aoun H**. When a house officer gets AIDS. N Engl J Med. 1989; 321:693-6.
8. **Zuger A, Miles SH. AIDS and Occupational Risk.** Historic traditions and ethical obligations. JAMA. 1987; 258:1924-8.
9. **Centers for Disease Control.** Guidelines for the prevention of transmission of Human Immunodeficiency Virus and Hepatitis B Virus to Health-Care and Public-Safety Workers. MMWR. 1989; 38:S-6.
10. **ACP Task Force on Adult Immunization and Infectious Diseases Society of America.** Guide for Adult Immunization (2nd ed.). Philadelphia, PA: American College of Physicians, 1990.
11. **Rizzo JA, Marder WD, Willke RJ.** Physician contact with and attitudes toward HIV-seropositive patients. Results from a national survey. Med Care. 1990; 28:251-60.

Ethics Case Study: The Dilemma of Dealing with an Impaired Colleague

Case History

Paul Daniels, MD, is an associate professor of medicine at General Hospital. He is well known for his clinical and diagnostic skills, and sees many patients who are referred to him because their cases are clinical "puzzles." He has been at General Hospital for 10 years, through internship and residency, and is respected within the institution.

Carla Martin, MD, is a recently appointed assistant professor of medicine at General Hospital. At a Saturday faculty party, Dr. Martin notices Dr. Daniels slurring his words and staggering; she is concerned about Dr. Daniels driving home while intoxicated. He assures her that he is sober and can drive safely.

During this conversation, Dr. Daniels' beeper goes off, and he answers his page. Dr. Martin overhears the discussion between Dr. Daniels and a new intern, and realizes that Dr. Daniels is on call. She hears Dr. Daniels prescribe an unusually large dose of digoxin for the patient in question. When Dr. Martin asks Dr. Daniels about the patient, he says the problem was routine and that the new intern had Julyitis.

Dr. Martin worries all weekend about the patient on digoxin. Monday morning, she finds the patient and reviews the chart. The intern had not followed Dr. Daniels' instructions and had given the patient a much lower dose. Dr. Martin tracks down the intern and asks about the digoxin dosage. The young intern says that she checked with a more senior resident because she thought she misheard Dr. Daniels' directions, and had given the lower dosage upon the resident's instructions. Dr. Martin assures the apologetic intern that she gave the patient the correct dosage, but does not tell her about Dr. Daniels' mistake.

That day, Dr. Martin tries to discuss the issue with Dr. Daniels, who tells her that she is completely out of line. He denies any inappropriate behavior or having a drinking problem. He questions Dr. Martin's motives and tells her to mind her own business.

Dr. Martin makes discreet inquiries about Dr. Daniels and discovers that other faculty members have noticed him drinking excessively at parties. In fact, his friends on the staff often draw straws to decide who will drive him home after a party. No one seems to be concerned about Dr. Daniels' clinical competence. As Dr. Martin decides what to do, she looks into programs at General Hospital for employees with substance abuse problems. She finds that General Hospital has had a voluntary, confidential program in place for 10 years. When a physician is involved, an immediate assessment is made of the physician's clinical competence and threat to patient safety. Clinical performance is monitored directly each week.

Dr. Martin is unsure about her next steps. Being relatively new to General Hospital, she questions her interpretation of Dr. Daniels' behavior. Other faculty members, who have known Dr. Daniels for a long time, seem unconcerned about his drinking. What should she do?

Commentary

This case study highlights the difficult issues surrounding the professional mandate to protect patients from physicians impaired by psychiatric, physiological or physical disorders. The *ACP Ethics Manual* is unequivocal: "It is the responsibility of every physician to protect the public from an impaired physician. . . . All steps must be taken to assure that no patient is harmed because of actions or decisions made by an impaired physician" (1). But upholding this duty often necessitates making a judgment about a colleague's impairment, as well as confronting institutional, social and personal barriers.

In this case study, Dr. Martin has direct evidence that a patient could have been harmed by Dr. Daniels' actions. She might not be in the best position to judge the level of his impairment, since she has limited experience with Dr. Daniels and in the institution. Nevertheless, it is her moral duty to ensure that his impairment and clinical competence are assessed by an appropriate authority.

Given that General Hospital has a voluntary, confidential program, it is best to confront Dr. Daniels again and ask him to seek help. If he refuses, Dr. Martin must inform the appropriate parties within the institution (possibly the division or department chief) about the incident she witnessed and her conversation with the young intern. If the institutional authorities fail to act, Dr. Martin should consider reporting Dr. Daniels to the state medical society (most societies have impaired physician programs).

We can envision the dilemmas facing Dr. Martin as she tries to fulfill her obligations. In General Hospital, Dr. Daniels is respected, well-known and tenured; Dr. Martin is a relatively new faculty member whose future at the hospital could be at stake. She might also have a normal aversion to confrontation, especially about a topic as sensitive as physician impairment. She might worry about losing the respect and trust of her peers, and about the legal implications of making such an accusation. Clearly, Dr. Martin takes a certain risk, personally and professionally, by pursuing this issue.

But confronting Dr. Daniels, or reporting him, need not be seen exclusively in a negative light. Great progress has been made in the treatment of the impaired physician in the past 20 years, since the AMA produced its landmark report, "The Sick Physician." In 1973 the AMA adopted the program recommended in its report, which stressed the physician's ethical obligation to help impaired colleagues while ensuring that impaired physicians do not endanger patients (2). Most programs now emphasize treatment and rehabilitation, rather than discipline and sanctions. And recovery rates for physicians are higher than the general population: in a case/control study, 83% of physicians had returned to practice and were functioning well three years after treatment, compared with 62% of middle-class control subjects (3).

Dr. Martin may also worry about her legal duties and protection. While statutes vary from state to state, many states have instituted "snitch laws" that require certain groups of people (such as physician colleagues and health care entities) to report knowledge of physician impairment to either a state medical society or licensing board (4).

Most laws provide a certain degree of anonymity for reporting parties as well as immunity from a civil suit, while setting penalties for those designated who do not report an impaired physician. Most laws also allow the impaired physician's records to remain confidential. However, Dr. Martin should contact her state medical society to find out the legal requirements in her state.

Regardless of Dr. Martin's legal duties, she is morally required to protect patients from harm. She must resist a natural impulse to avoid maligning a colleague, especially a senior one, or to identify with Dr. Daniels (there but for the grace of God . . .). Certainly, she should act carefully and discreetly, but she must also take definitive actions.

How far does Dr. Martin's obligation extend? If Dr. Daniels agrees to seek treatment, how can Dr. Martin be sure he goes? Is it even appropriate for her to check? If she reports Dr. Daniels to the department head, is her obligation fulfilled even if the department head fails to act? In other words, when has Dr. Martin done enough?

We do not see easy answers to these questions. There may be practical limits to what Dr. Martin can do within her institution and in her role as Dr. Daniels' colleague. One person cannot become completely responsible for the actions of another. However, it is reasonable to use the following rule as a guide: A physician's obligation corresponds to how much evidence exists that a patient could be harmed.

In our case study, Dr. Martin knows that a patient could have been harmed, and she should assume that Dr. Daniels' other patients are at risk. Thus, her obligation extends further than if she had only noticed Dr. Daniels drinking excessively at a party when he was not on call. In that case, it might have been sufficient to express her concern to Dr. Daniels only, and to remain alert to other signs of Dr. Daniels' potential impairment.

While we have emphasized Dr. Martin's ethical obligations here, we do not minimize Dr. Daniels' responsibility for his own behavior. He clearly violated the maxim, *primum non nocere*—"first, do no harm," which has been a cornerstone of physician ethics for centuries.

Beyond the direct threat to patient safety, Dr. Daniels' drinking could also have dire consequences for the young interns and residents he supervises.

Clearly, Dr. Daniels bears the ultimate responsibility for his impairment. But this acknowledgement should not obscure the nature of Dr. Daniels' problem, which is substance abuse. His improper actions are a result of a disease, and as such he deserves treatment, rather than discipline.

At every step, the ultimate goal of all parties—the impaired physician, knowing colleagues and institutional programs—is protection of patients, rehabilitation of the impaired physician and a return to clinical competence.

Acknowledgment: The Ethics Committee would like to thank Janet Weiner, MPH, primary author of this case history and commentary.

References

1. **American College of Physicians.** American College of Physicians Ethics Manual. Part 1: History; The Patient; Other Physicians. Ann Intern Med. 1989; 111:254-52; Part 2: The Physician and Society; Research: Life-Sustaining Treatment; Other Issues. Ann Intern Med. 1989; 111: 327-35.
2. **Sargent DA**. The impaired physician movement: An interim report. Hosp Comm Psychiatry. 1985; 36:294-7.
3. Ibid., p. 297.
4. **Walzer RS**. Impaired physicians: An overview and update of the legal issues. J Leg Med. 1990; 11:131-98.

Ethics Case Study: Ms. Washington Is Terminally Ill and Wants to Die—Should Dr. Jones Assist?

Case History

Ella Washington, age 60, visits Dr. Jones, her internist for the past 20 years, with complaints of nausea, stomach pain and weight loss. Dr. Jones' workup reveals pancreatic cancer, with metastases to the liver.

Dr. Jones and Ms. Washington talk extensively about the diagnosis, her poor prognosis and the lack of curative therapies. In response to her direct question, Dr. Jones says that Ms. Washington probably has less than six months to live. He refers her to an oncologist for further advice, and schedules another appointment with him a few weeks later to go over the situation.

Ms. Washington returns in a few weeks, accompanied by her husband and son. She has consulted the oncologist and seems to have a clear understanding of her condition. Her family appears supportive as they talk about palliative therapies and home hospice care.

Before leaving, Ms. Washington tells Dr. Jones that she wants to "die with dignity," and needs to be able to take her own life in the least painful way possible when the time comes. She says that she has spoken to her family at length and that they support her decision. She claims that fear of a painful, lingering death will prevent her from enjoying her remaining time. She tells Dr. Jones that she obtained information from the Hemlock Society on methods of suicide and bought a copy of "Final Exit" by the society's executive director. She asks Dr. Jones to prescribe barbiturates.

Dr. Jones initially refuses Ms. Washington's request, and asks her to return to see him in a few weeks after she consults with a psychiatrist to verify that she is not significantly depressed. She complies, and returns to Dr. Jones with the same prescription request. "This is my decision," she says firmly. "We've known each other a long time. I trust you; but if you don't help me, I'll find someone who will or do it myself. Please don't make this harder on me and my family."

She explains that the security of having enough barbiturates to commit suicide, when and if the time comes, would allow her to live fully and enjoy the present. Dr. Jones is convinced that Ms. Washington is not despondent and is thinking rationally. They agree to meet regularly, and she promises to consult with him before taking her life. Dr. Jones then writes the prescription for barbiturates.

The next four months are intense for Ms. Washington, and while she tires easily and has some pain, this is a fulfilling period. She spends time with her husband and son, and renews and reinforces old friendships. She endures intermittent physical and emotional hardships, but seems to bounce back from periods of sadness and anger.

But then she becomes weaker, and the nausea and stomach pain grow more constant and intense. Despite extensive efforts to minimize her discomfort, she feels that the immediate future holds what she fears most: increased pain, dependence and disability. As agreed, she meets with Dr. Jones to inform him that she would soon commit suicide. Two days later, Ms. Washington's husband calls to say that she died at home, after saying goodbye to her family and closest friends.

Commentary

Background

When Jack Kevorkian, MD, enabled Janet Adkins to end her life last year using the "suicide machine" he had set up in his Volkswagen van, attention centered on the fact that Dr. Kevorkian did not have a longstanding doctor-patient relationship with the Alzheimer's disease victim, was not involved in her current care, was not specially trained in assessing depression, and Mrs. Adkins was not terminally ill.

These issues, though important, deflected discussion from what should have been a prior question, the question so sharply brought into focus by the case detailed in this article, but common to both cases: May a physician ever ethically assist a patient who wishes to commit suicide? Thousands of years of medical ethics tradition has said no. The Hippocratic Oath says no: "I will give no deadly medicine to anyone if asked, nor suggest any such counsel." More recently, ACP's *Ethics Manual* has said no: "Although a patient may refuse a medical intervention and the physician may comply with this refusal, the physician must never intentionally and directly cause death or assist a patient to commit suicide" (1). The AMA has said no. "In assisted suicide . . . the primary purpose of the treatment is to cause death. And that purpose has no role in the professional responsibilities of the physician" (2).

A distinguished panel of physicians, however, recently concluded that "it is not immoral for a physician to assist in the rational suicide of a terminally ill person" (3). And advances in medical technology and compelling cases such as that of Dr. Jones and Ms. Washington in this article require us to look at these issues anew.

Withholding or withdrawing life-sustaining treatment, physician-assisted suicide and active euthanasia form a spectrum of issues in end-of-life decision-making. Much has been said about the distinctions between forgoing life-sustaining treatment and euthanasia. This commentary, instead, will focus on assisted suicide.

Conflicting 'Goods'

There have always been people who have wanted medicine—through assisted suicide or euthanasia—to help bring about their deaths. That has not changed. Medicine's ability to prolong the dying process in certain circumstances has increased, as has its ability to relieve pain. Not all patients, however, have access to appropriate pain management and supportive care. This may lead some to see suicide as their only option.

Good hospice-type care should be a high priority for all patients. Even though most patients who receive it find that quality terminal care meets their needs, a few, like Ms. Washington, want more control.

The "no's" listed earlier in this commentary reflect the fundamental tenet of medicine that physicians be and be seen as healers and comforters, not agents of death. When physicians cannot heal, however, is life to be sustained at all costs? For example, many physicians agree that once the diagnosis is confirmed, it is not unethical to withdraw the life support of a patient in a persistent vegetative state, based on patient wishes.

Is there, as has traditionally been thought, a clear distinction between omitting care at a patient's request that may or may not result in death, and actively and intentionally causing (or assisting to cause) death? Between giving someone the means to end his or her own life and directly ending a life? The preservation of life, the restoration of health, the relief of suffering and respect for patient autonomy—these four "goods" sometimes conflict. How should they be balanced?

Here, Dr. Jones wants nothing more than to do what is best for a terminally ill patient for whom he has cared for 20 years. He fears the possibility of a botched suicide attempt. Knowing that she does not have much time, Ms. Washington has a clear conception of how she wants to live the remainder of her life. Ms. Washington and Dr. Jones were ultimately able to discuss her views and wishes openly.

In deciding to comply with his patient's wishes, Dr. Jones is doing what he believes will relieve her current and anticipated suffering. In addition, he might say he looked to the principle of patient autonomy as his guide in determining to honor Ms. Washington's request. Ms. Washington had no interest in testing further modern medicine's ability to relieve pain and understood that her strength could not be restored. She foresaw what she believed would soon be a life of increased pain, dependence and disability.

Sanctity of Life

Physicians are charged to "do no harm." Is there something objectively harmful, or harmful in the eyes of society, about assisting suicide? Ms. Washington maintains that harm will only come to her if Dr. Jones does not help her to live out her remaining time with the peace of mind that will come if she can choose death. She is appealing to Dr. Jones to relieve suffering as she defines it. Can harm be done when a person does not acknowledge or recognize it?

Under a "sanctity of human life" argument, the answer would be yes. Whether based in religion or on the belief that this principle provides a foundation for social order, "sanctity of life" dictates that life is sacred and should not be taken. But what about exceptions to the rule? Should physician-assisted suicide ever be one?

'Slippery Slopes' and Other Arguments

Those opposing physician-assisted suicide argue further that the potential consequences of such a practice could have additional adverse effects on health care: "The dedication of the medical profession to the welfare of patients and to the promotion of their health might be seriously undermined in the eyes of the public and of patients by the complicity of physicians in the death of the very ill" (4). Also, providing suicide assistance could compromise patient trust in physicians (2).

But like "slippery slope" arguments, these positions do not address whether it is ever ethical for physicians to provide suicide assistance so much as call attention to the need for rigorous procedures to safeguard patient rights if assistance was to be sanctioned.

This leads us to slippery slope arguments. Even if in an individual case—assisting the suicide of a thoughtful, emotionally prepared terminally ill patient such as Ms. Washington—might seem benevolent, what would be the social consequences of the acceptance of this practice? Would patients come to feel they have a "duty" to die? Would this lead to more active and less voluntary forms of euthanasia? What about the risk of error and opportunities for abuse?

These questions are certainly legitimate but again, it may well be that they could be satisfactorily addressed by carefully constructed procedures and some kind of oversight of the assisted suicide process. The primary question is, are there circumstances under which it would be ethical for a physician to provide assistance?

More Unanswered Questions

More questions remain unanswered: Are some patients requesting assisted suicide because they fear that they will not be allowed to refuse life support when the time comes? Conversely, would demands for assisted suicide create a backlash that would make it more difficult to withhold or withdraw life-sustaining treatment? If assisted suicide were to become accepted, would physicians have less incentive to optimize supportive care?

Public interest in the issue of physician-assisted suicide is deep and pervasive. Opinion polls suggest that about equal numbers favor and oppose it. Clearly the profession as well as society need to continue to discuss the topic and to try to agree on public and professional policy.

In the meantime, physicians cannot be compelled to assist a suicide. And in considering or acting on these issues, physicians should remember that what they consider ethical may conflict with criminal or civil law, which varies from state to state. Physicians may wish to consult with local counsel before taking actions that may have legal consequences for themselves, their patients and their patients' families.

The Future

The practice of medicine has implications far beyond the examining room. The Hippocratic precept "first, do no harm" today involves harm done to the patient's rights, as well as to his or her welfare. Respect for patient autonomy, a hallmark of modern biomedical ethics, dictates that physicians uphold the informed treatment decisions of competent patients. But the profession's ethical integrity and medicine's obligations to society are threatened when a patient requests the assistance of medicine in order to commit suicide.

Perhaps what is driving the renewed debate about physician-assisted suicide is the rise of patient autonomy seen in the treatment refusal context. It is a settled question that adult patients (or their surrogates) retain authority for decision-making about health care. But how to define the range of patient decisions that physicians should comply with, and whether requests for physician-assisted suicide fit into that range, is unresolved.

Should physician-assisted suicide be permissible under certain circumstances, a next step beyond the withdrawal of feeding tubes and respirators? Or should it be forbidden under all circumstances? The profession and society need to decide.

Acknowledgments: The Ethics Committee would like to thank Janet Weiner, MPH, and Lois Snyder, JD, primary authors of this case history and commentary, respectively. Comments, as well as suggestions for future case studies, may be sent to Ms. Snyder in the Scientific Policy Department at ACP Headquarters.

References

1. **Ethics Committee, American College of Physicians**. American College of Physicians Ethics Manual. Part 2. Ann Intern Med. 1989; 111:327-35.
2. **Orentlicher D**. Physician participation in assisted suicide. JAMA. 1989; 262:1844-5, citing "Report of the Council on Ethical and Judicial Affairs of the American Medical Association: Euthanasia." Chicago, Ill.: American Medical Association; 1989.

3. **Wanzer SH, Federman DD, Adelstein SJ, et al.** The physician's responsibility toward hopelessly ill patients: A second look. N Engl J Med. 1989; 320:844-9.
4. **Jonsen AR, Siegler M, Winslade WJ**. "Clinical Ethics." New York: Macmillan Publishing Co., 1986.

Ethics Case Study: Does a Doctor-Patient Relationship Always Rule Out Sex?

Case History

Leonard Sullivan, MD, 59, has been one of three general internists in Pumpkin Hills, Wyo., for the past 30 years. He came to Pumpkin Hills immediately after residency, married a local woman and raised two children, now away at college. Dr. Sullivan's wife died of breast cancer one year ago.

Margaret Dinardo, 60, has spent her life in Pumpkin Hills, and has been a patient of Dr. Sullivan's for nearly 20 years. Her husband died two years ago, and her children are now married with families of their own.

Ms. Dinardo returns for her yearly visit with Dr. Sullivan. He finds her in continued good health, renews her Feldene prescription for mild osteoarthritis, and schedules her yearly mammogram. Dr. Sullivan reviews the results of his clinical exam, and they talk about general preventive health measures. He notices that he feels uplifted by Ms. Dinardo's presence.

"Enough about me, Leonard," Ms. Dinardo says finally. "How have you been since Diane passed on?"

"It's been difficult, although the children have been a great help," he responds. Ms. Dinardo touches his shoulder, saying, "I know exactly what you mean," and leaves. About a week later, Ms. Dinardo calls Dr. Sullivan at home and invites him over for dinner. "I bet you don't get many home-cooked meals these days," she says. He accepts, and they spend the evening talking. Dr. Sullivan tells her about his life now, and the trouble he has had coping with the death of his wife. In Margaret Dinardo, he finds an understanding and compassionate listener, who shares her experiences since losing her spouse. "Thank you, Margaret . . . I feel so much better talking to you," he says.

"Any time, Leonard," she responds. "Call me and maybe we'll catch a movie."

In the next few months, Dr. Sullivan and Ms. Dinardo see each other regularly. They enjoy each other's company and consider their relationship to be an evolution of their longstanding friendship. But Dr. Sullivan begins to notice that he feels romantically inclined toward Ms. Dinardo, and wonders if she feels the same way. One evening, Ms. Dinardo says, "Leonard, what is the matter with you? You've been fidgeting since you got here." He blurts out that he feels attracted to her romantically, and she replies, "Well, it's about time! I was beginning to think you were just too old for me!"

They kiss passionately, well into the evening. He reluctantly draws away from her and heads toward the door. "I really should be getting home. . . . I have a busy day tomorrow at the office. Good night, Margaret."

"Oh well, your duty calls. Good night, Dr. Sullivan," she replies.

He does not sleep at all, feeling strangely disquieted by the word "doctor." All day, he is troubled by Ms. Dinardo's use of "Dr. Sullivan." After a long day at the office, he decides to talk to her about it. "You know, I was always taught that a sexual relationship between a doctor and a patient was wrong," he begins. "If we're going to start something here, maybe you should consider becoming Dr. Voorhees' patient."

Ms. Dinardo reacts with surprise and anger. "Leonard Sullivan, you have been my doctor for 20 years. I trust you—that doesn't just go away because we kissed. How can you even think such a thing?" She refuses to consider seeing another internist. "Listen, we kissed yesterday, and you expect me to give you up as a doctor? You must be kidding!"

What should Dr. Sullivan do?

Commentary

This case study illustrates some of the subtleties and difficulties inherent in the general prohibition against sex between doctor and patient. The prohibition dates back to at least the Hippocratic Oath, which states, "I will come for the benefit of the sick, remaining free of all intentional injustice, of all mischief and in particular of sexual relations with both male and female persons . . . " (1). Although medical and ethical consensus on the prohibition remains intact, recently publicized abuses have brought renewed public and professional attention to the issue.

The upcoming edition of ACP's *Ethics Manual* is clear on this point: "It is unethical for a physician to become sexually involved with a current patient even if the patient initiates or consents to the advances." Likewise, the AMA concludes that "sexual contact or a romantic relationship with a patient concurrent with the physician-patient relationship is unethical" (2). Both sources also question the wisdom of sexual relationships with former patients. The AMA and ACP consider it unethical "if the physician uses or exploits trust, knowledge, emotions or influence derived from the previous professional relationship."

In reaching its recommendation against sexual contact between physicians and patients, the ACP Ethics Committee considered four arguments:

- **The inequality between the parties.** In doctor-patient relationships, patients answer personal questions, reveal sensitive information and allow the doctor to touch them. This is one-way intimacy; doctors do not ordinarily put themselves in similar positions. True consent by the patient to an intimate relationship is questionable, and initiation of one suspect, given this inequality.
- **The inherent vulnerability of the patient.** Most patients seeking care are ill, and put great faith in the doctor's opinion and advice. The inequality in knowledge and health status puts patients in a vulnerable and dependent position, one that physicians must never exploit.
- **The possibility of betraying the patient's trust.** The social contract between physicians and patients is based on trust; patients trust that the doctor will keep all information confidential, and will only use such information to help them. At some point in an intimate relationship, a doctor might use knowledge gained from the therapeutic relationship out of self-interest, or a patient or community might perceive this to be the case. This undermines trust in the profession as a whole.
- **The conflict with the physician's duty to act in the patient's best interests.** In the therapeutic relationship, patients trust that the doctor will keep their interests primary. In a sexual relationship, there are competing and sometimes conflicting interests. The two relationships cannot be reconciled.

For these reasons, we believe that sex between doctors and current patients is unethical. Our ethical concerns are mirrored in legal and regulatory sanctions against this practice. The laws of a number of states consider sexual contact between physicians and patients to be criminal behavior, and such contact is almost universally grounds for action by state licensing boards.

In many ways, our case is not typical of sexual misconduct by doctors who abuse their patients. This is a reality we do not mean to ignore or diminish by the case we have presented. For example, cases of an obstetrician raping a patient under anesthesia, or a psychiatrist having sex with a patient under the guise of therapy, are so obviously wrong that the ethics need no explanation. To explore whether the professional ethic holds true in less obvious situations, we have deliberately crafted the most benign, longstanding physician-patient relationship we could imagine.

Despite prohibitions, we find that 5%-10% of all psychiatrists report sexual contact with a patient, and it is likely that these figures hold true for other specialists (3). Most of this contact appears clearly exploitative of the patient within the therapeutic relationship. There are well-documented reports of harm to patients from these relationships, which can have devastating effects on their lives and their capacity to trust any other physician. In published studies, 85%-90% of patients experience sexual contact with their physician as damaging, although the data may be biased by selective reporting of more negative reactions (4). Female patients (overwhelmingly the objects of such contact) have been reported to experience guilt, severe distrust of their own judgment and mistrust of both men and physicians.

We turn now to the more difficult case, like our Dr. Sullivan, in which the physician and patient find themselves attracted to one another in a relationship concurrent with, but apart from, the therapeutic relationship. This can be especially a problem within small rural communities, where a large proportion of the community may be the physician's patients.

On the surface, our case lacks many of the aspects that make physician-patient sex so disconcerting: Ms. Dinardo does not seem especially vulnerable, since she is not acutely or chronically ill. Dr. Sullivan does not seem to be betraying Ms. Dinardo's trust, and their relationship does not seem unequal. Indeed, they seem to step out of their roles in the social context in which they continue to see each other. Should this kind of situation be considered just a matter of consensual activity between two adults? Does the ethical prohibition apply, and if so, why?

In our case, the dangers are subtle but still present. Twenty years of a therapeutic relationship may have produced a dependence in Ms. Dinardo that Dr. Sullivan does not recognize. Indeed, Dr. Sullivan's ready willingness to transfer Ms. Dinardo's care, and her extreme objection to being transferred, point to a difference in both perception and power. Physicians and patients may view the sexual relationship quite differently as well, and not share the same understanding of the effect of their ongoing or previous therapeutic relationship.

If Dr. Sullivan tries to maintain dual relationships, he would violate a fundamental tenet of medical ethics and physician practice—the promise to keep his patient's interests primary. This violation would occur regardless of the outcome of their intimate relationship. In a sexual relationship, Dr. Sullivan necessarily elevates his own interests to at least the same level as his patient's. He begins to act in his own best interest. Perhaps these interests converge with his patient's, and they will live happily ever after. In that case, Dr. Sullivan's objectivity would be colored, and we would recommend that he not continue to take care of Ms. Dinardo, for many of the same reasons physicians should not provide ongoing medical care to family members.

But there is no guarantee of future happiness. One of the strongest arguments against physician-patient sex is that it might not work out forever. Dr. Sullivan and Ms. Dinardo could embark upon an intimate relationship that falls apart after a length of time. Perhaps the breakup would not be without rancor. It is likely that Dr. Sullivan and Ms. Dinardo could not continue a trusting doctor-patient relationship, and one or both would want to sever the professional ties. In that scenario, it is clearer that the patient's interests had not remained primary, and had led to a conflict of interest.

Therefore, in either scenario, it would not be in Ms. Dinardo's best interests to remain Dr. Sullivan's patient if they want to become more intimate. It would also not be in Dr. Sullivan's best interests. He risks losing his license if reported to the state board, and risks the confidence of his other patients and the community if he becomes intimate with a current patient. Knowing this, it is important to transfer her care before they begin an intimate relationship.

Even former patients may continue to feel dependent or vulnerable, and Dr. Sullivan should carefully assess this possibility (and consultation with an objective colleague may help). The danger to former patients of psychiatrists has been recognized by criminal or civil laws in a number of states (5). Most of these laws dictate a one- to two-year interval as an appropriate safeguard against abuse. Of course, internists may not face the same issues of transference and power imbalance as psychiatrists. We believe that the delay necessary to protect a patient will vary with the people involved and the nature, extent and intensity of the prior professional relationship.

And so we return to the question posed in our case: What should Dr. Sullivan do about Ms. Dinardo and their growing romantic involvement?

Acknowledgment: The Ethics Committee would like to thank Janet Weiner, MPH, and Susan Tolle, FACP, primary authors of this case history and commentary.

References

1. **Council on Ethical and Judicial Affairs, American Medical Association**. Sexual misconduct in the practice of medicine. JAMA. 1991; 266:2741-5.
2. Ibid., p. 2745.
3. **Gartrell N, Herman J, Olarte S, Feldstein M, Localio R**. Psychiatrist-patient sexual contact: Results of a national survey, I: Prevalence. Am J Psychiatry. 1986; 143:1126-31.
4. **Council on Ethical and Judicial Affairs, American Medical Association**. Sexual misconduct in the practice of medicine. JAMA. 1991; 266:2741-5.
5. **Applebaum PS, Jorgenson L**. Psychotherapist-patient sexual contact after termination of treatment: An analysis and a proposal. Am J Psychiatry. 1991; 148:1466-73.